Multiple Choice Questions in

INTENSIVE CARE MEDICINE

Steve Benington
Peter Nightingale
Maire Shelly

tfm Publishing Limited, Castle Hill Barns, Harley, Nr Shrewsbury, SY5 6LX, UK. Tel: +44 (0)1952 510061; Fax: +44 (0)1952 510192 E-mail: nikki@tfmpublishing.com; Web site: www.tfmpublishing.com

Design & Typesetting: Nikki Bramhill BSc Hons Dip Law
First Edition: © 2009
Paperback   ISBN: 978-1-903378-64-9
Reprinted December 2010, December 2013, January 2021

E-book editions: 2014
ePub   ISBN: 978-1-908986-36-8
Mobi   ISBN: 978-1-908986-37-5
Web pdf   ISBN: 978-1-908986-38-2

Printed by Gutenberg Press Ltd., Gudja Road, Tarxien, PLA 19, Malta. Tel: +356 21897037; Fax: +356 21800069.

Contents

Preface

While preparing recently for the multiple choice component of the European Diploma in Intensive Care (EDIC), I was struck by the fact that there were no dedicated MCQ books available to aid my revision. While intensive care medicine has long formed part of the syllabus for professional examinations in anaesthesia, surgery and medicine in the UK, various standalone qualifications (including the European and UK diplomas) are now available. While currently 'desirable', their possession is likely to become mandatory in the near future for senior trainees; MCQs will remain a tried and tested means of assessing the candidate's knowledge.

The 300 MCQs herein are intended to cover the breadth of knowledge required of the practising intensive care physician. They draw on the Competency-Based Training programme in Intensive Care Medicine (CoBaTrICE) syllabus provided by the European Society of Intensive Care Medicine. Topics include resuscitation, diagnosis, disease management, practical procedures, peri-operative care, ethics and applied basic science. The answer to each question is accompanied by short referenced notes sourced from peer-reviewed journals, educational articles and major critical care textbooks.

I hope this book will be of value not only to those preparing for professional examinations in the specialty, but also to junior intensive care trainees and senior intensive care nurses wishing to expand their knowledge, and to practising intensive care physicians as a teaching aid. In addition, trainees in the specialties mentioned above may also find this book a useful complement to their exam preparation.

I would like to thank both editors, Maire Shelly and Peter Nightingale, for their time and invaluable help in preparing this manuscript. Both are busy intensive care physicians with regional and national responsibilities, and both are EDIC examiners with a major commitment to teaching and training. Many of the questions in this book have been rewritten, had ambiguities removed or been otherwise honed as a result of their careful scrutiny; any remaining errors are my responsibility.

Steve Benington MB ChB MRCP FRCA, *Specialist Registrar*
Anaesthesia & Intensive Care Medicine, Manchester, UK
February 2009

Foreword

This book marks the beginning of an era! Intensive care medicine is not only included in books of MCQs in anaesthesia, surgery and medicine, it now has a specialty-based MCQ book in its own right.

MCQs are now a fact of life for those sitting undergraduate and postgraduate medical examinations. To be successful it is essential that candidates have a sound knowledge base and practise their technique adequately beforehand. This collection of MCQs has been put together by Dr Steve Benington primarily as an aid for those sitting the European Diploma of Intensive Care (EDIC) but its appeal will undoubtedly be wider. Members of the multidisciplinary team on the ICU, those in other specialties who wish to expand their knowledge and trainers who are helping candidates to prepare for the examination, will all find it invaluable.

It has been our privilege to help him develop this book. We hope the material within will act as a useful guide to the scope and standard of the EDIC and will inspire others to learn more about intensive care medicine.

Peter Nightingale FRCA FRCP
Consultant in Anaesthesia & Intensive Care Medicine
Intensive Care Unit, Wythenshawe Hospital
Manchester, UK

Maire Shelly MB ChB FRCA
Consultant in Anaesthesia & Intensive Care Medicine
Intensive Care Unit, Wythenshawe Hospital
Manchester, UK

February 2009

Abbreviations

ACS:	Abdominal compartment syndrome
AF:	Atrial fibrillation
AFLP:	Acute fatty liver of pregnancy
AG:	Anion gap
AIS:	Abbreviated Injury Scale
ALI:	Acute lung injury
ALT:	Alanine aminotransferase
APACHE:	Acute Physiology And Chronic Health Evaluation
APTT:	Activated partial thromboplastin time
ARDS:	Acute respiratory distress syndrome
ARF:	Acute renal failure
AST:	Aspartate aminotransferase
ATLS®:	Advanced Trauma Life Support
ATP:	Adenosine triphosphate
AV:	Atrioventricular
AVNRT:	Atrioventricular non-re-entrant tachycardias
AVRTs:	Atrioventricular re-entrant tachycardias
BOOP:	Bronchiolitis obliterans organising pneumonia
BP:	Blood pressure
bpm:	Beats per minute
BSA:	Body surface area
BUN:	Blood urea nitrogen
CAM-ICU:	Confusion Assessment Method for ICU patients
CIP:	Critical illness polyneuromyopathy
CMV:	Continuous mandatory ventilation
COPD:	Chronic obstructive pulmonary disease
CPAP:	Continuous positive airway pressure
CPP:	Cerebral perfusion pressure
CRRT:	Continuous renal replacement therapy
CSF:	Cerebrospinal fluid
CVP:	Central venous pressure
CVVH:	Continuous veno-venous haemofiltration
CXR:	Chest x-ray
DIC:	Disseminated intravascular coagulation
DOCS:	Disorders of Consciousness Scale
DVT:	Deep vein thrombosis
ECG:	Electrocardiogram

EMF:	Electromotive force
ESBL:	Extended spectrum ß-lactamase
ESR:	Erythrocyte sedimentation rate
EVLW:	Extravascular lung water
FAST:	Focused abdominal ultrasound for trauma
FEV1:	Forced expiratory volume in 1 second
FFP:	Fresh frozen plama
FTc:	Flow time (corrected)
GABA:	Gamma-hydroxybutyric acid
GCS:	Glasgow Coma Scale
GEDV:	Global end-diastolic volume
GFR:	Glomerular filtration rate
GHB:	Gamma-hydroxybutyrate
HbF:	Foetal haemoglobin
HELLP:	Haemolysis, elevated liver enzymes and low platelets
HFOV:	High-frequency oscillatory ventilation
HR:	Heart rate
HSE:	*Herpes simplex* encephalitis
IABP:	Intra-aortic balloon pump
ICP:	Intracranial pressure
ICU:	Intensive care unit
IHCA:	In-hospital cardiac arrest
IHD:	Ischaemic heart disease
INR:	International normalised ratio
IPF:	Idiopathic pulmonary fibrosis
ISS:	Injury Severity Score
JVP:	Jugular venous pressure
LVAD:	Left ventricular assist device
LVEDP:	Left ventricular end-diastolic pressure
MAP:	Mean arterial pressure
MG:	Myasthenia gravis
MI:	Myocardial infarction
MRSA:	Methicillin-resistant *Staphylococcus aureus*
MS:	Multiple sclerosis
NAC:	N-acetylcysteine
NSAID:	Non-steroidal anti-inflammatory drug
NSTEMI:	Non-ST-segment-elevation myocardial infarction
OHCA:	Out-of-hospital cardiac arrest
PAOP:	Pulmonary artery occlusion pressure
PCI:	Percutaneous coronary intervention
PCP:	Phencyclidine

PCR:	Polymerase chain reaction
PE:	Pulmonary embolism
PEA:	Pulseless electrical activity
PEEP:	Positive end-expiratory pressure
PET:	Positron emission tomography
PT:	Prothrombin time
PTS:	Post-traumatic seizures
PVS:	Persistent vegetative state
rFVIIa:	Recombinant factor VIIa
rhAPC:	Recombinant human activated protein C
ROSC:	Return of spontaneous circulation
RR:	Respiratory rate
RRT:	Renal replacement therapy
RV:	Residual volume
SA:	Sino-atrial
SAPS:	Simplified Acute Physiology Scores
SDH:	Subdural haematoma
SIADH:	Syndrome of inappropriate antidiuretic hormone secretion
SIRS:	Systemic inflammatory response syndrome
SLE:	Systemic lupus erythematosus
SOFA:	Sequential Organ Failure Assessment
SpO_2:	Oxygen saturation by pulse oximetry
SRMD:	Stress-related mucosal damage
SSRI:	Serotonin reuptake inhibitor
STEMI:	ST-elevation myocardial infarction
SV:	Stroke volume
SVR:	Systemic vascular resistance
TBI:	Traumatic brain injury
TLC:	Total lung capacity
TPA:	Tissue plasminogen activator
TPN:	Total parenteral nutrition
TRALI:	Transfusion-related acute lung injury
TRH:	Thyrotrophin releasing hormone
TSH:	Thyroid stimulating hormone
TXA:	Tranexamic acid
VAP:	Ventilator-associated pneumonia
VCD:	Vocal cord dysfunction
Vd:	Volume of distribution
VF:	Ventricular fibrillation
VTE:	Venous thromboembolism
WPW:	Wolff-Parkinson-White

How to use this book

Answering the questions

This book contains three 100-question multiple choice papers. Each paper comprises 50 Type 'A' and 50 Type 'K' questions, following the format of the EDIC Part 1 examination. There is no negative marking and therefore every question should be attempted. Under exam conditions a maximum time of three hours is permitted to complete a paper.

Type 'A' questions require the candidate to select the SINGLE best answer from the five options presented. In some cases the other four options are clearly wrong, but in others the distinction will be less clear-cut. The accompanying referenced notes should clarify the reasoning behind the correct answer.

Type 'K' questions consist of a statement followed by four stems, EACH requiring a 'True' or 'False' answer.

Marking the questions

The maximum score for a paper is 100 marks. For Type 'A' questions 1 mark is scored for a correct answer, and 0 for a wrong answer. For Type 'K' questions 1 mark is scored if all four stems are answered correctly, with a half mark if three out of four are correct. No marks are scored if more than one stem is answered incorrectly.

For the EDIC part I examination, the pass mark is set based on the mean and standard deviation of the marks of candidates in any one sitting. Previously this has been around 55-60%. The questions in this book are intended to be of a similar level of difficulty. A candidate scoring over 60% can be confident that they are well-prepared, while a score of 50% or below means further work is required!

Paper 1

Type 'A' questions

A1 Regarding electrolyte administration in the adult the following are true EXCEPT:

a. Infusion of potassium should not normally exceed 40mmol/h.
b. Daily sodium requirement is 1-2mmol/kg.
c. Most calcium in the extracellular fluid is protein-bound.
d. 1g of magnesium sulphate contains 4mmol magnesium.
e. The normal range for phosphate in the plasma is 0.8-1.5mmol/L (2.5-4.6mg/dL).

A2 The following ECG is compatible with a diagnosis of:

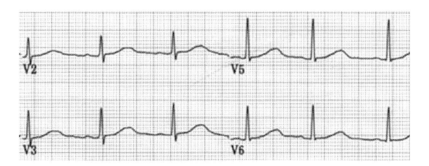

a. Hyperkalaemia.
b. Hypocalcaemia.
c. Hypothermia.
d. Acute anterolateral myocardial infarction.
e. Hyponatraemia.

A3   The following reduce the risk of electrical injury in the ICU EXCEPT:

a.   Mains isolating transformer.
b.   Earth leakage circuit breaker.
c.   Use of a common earth.
d.   Ensuring the patient has a good earth connection.
e.   Use of Class II equipment.

A4   Which of the following is NOT an effective (>1°C/h fall in temperature) method of inducing therapeutic hypothermia in an ICU patient?

a.   Cold air blanket.
b.   Ice water bodily immersion.
c.   Extracorporeal heat exchange.
d.   Rapid infusion of 30ml/kg bolus of crystalloid at 4°C.
e.   Central venous cooling catheter.

A5   A 38-year-old window cleaner falls from the fifth floor of a building. On arrival in the Emergency Room, his Glasgow Coma Score (GCS) is 15 and he complains of pain, with bruising, of his chest wall. He also has a fractured left distal tibia and fibula. Blood pressure (BP) is 80/40mmHg, heart rate (HR) is 130bpm and respiratory rate (RR) is 30 breaths per minute. The CXR shows a small right-sided pulmonary contusion and a sternal fracture. The ECG shows right bundle branch block and T-wave inversion in V1. Despite rapid infusion of 3L of crystalloid his blood pressure falls to 60/40mmHg and his heart rate increases further. Insertion of bilateral chest drains has no effect. Abdominal ultrasound shows no evidence of free fluid. The MOST LIKELY diagnosis is:

a.   Extensive pulmonary contusion.
b.   Cardiac tamponade.
c.   Myocardial infarction.
d.   Fat embolism.
e.   Ruptured spleen.

A6   A 22-year-old man is being observed in the ICU following an incident where he was stabbed in the left flank. He was initially haemodynamically stable, but deteriorates several hours later, becoming pale and clammy with a HR of 125bpm, RR of 26 breaths per minute and BP of 78/58mmHg. His chest X-ray shows no abnormality. Regarding the immediate resuscitation of this patient which ONE of the following is TRUE?

a.   Human albumin 4% will be no more effective than crystalloid for fluid resuscitation.
b.   Blood substitutes should be used in preference to crystalloid for initial resuscitation if available.
c.   Level 1 evidence supports the use of hypotensive resuscitation in this setting.
d.   A transfusion trigger of 7-9g/dl should be used.
e.   A central venous catheter should be placed immediately to guide further fluid therapy.

A7   A 55-year-old woman is thrown from a motorbike during a collision and is found unresponsive at the roadside by the paramedics. On arrival in the Emergency Room she is haemodynamically stable; BP is 131/74mmHg, HR is 85bpm, RR is 8 breaths per minute and SpO_2 is 98% on 15L of oxygen via a non-rebreathing mask. Her GCS is 6 and she has a dilated unreactive left pupil. Following rapid sequence induction of anaesthesia and tracheal intubation, a CT brain scan shows normal brain parenchyma with blood in the lateral ventricles. She is transferred to the ICU for further management. The following are adverse prognostic factors EXCEPT:

a.   Female gender.
b.   Her age.
c.   A dilated unreactive pupil.
d.   Her GCS after resuscitation.
e.   Subarachnoid blood on CT scan.

A8   A 51-year-old homeless man is brought into hospital with a severe headache, neck stiffness and vomiting. He complains of a 6-week period of feeling 'rotten'. On examination he has opisthotonus, mild papilloedema and photophobia. He is drowsy and has a temperature of 37.9°C. Blood tests include a white cell count of 13x10^3/mL. Lumbar puncture shows clear cerebrospinal fluid (CSF) with a lymphocytic pleocytosis, protein 1g/L, glucose 1.5mmol/L (27.3mg/dL). India ink stain is negative. The most likely diagnosis is:

a.   Tuberculous meningitis.
b.   Viral meningitis.
c.   Pneumococcal meningitis.
d.   Cryptococcal meningitis.
e.   None of the above.

A9   Which statement regarding right ventricular infarction is FALSE?

a.   Right atrial pressure is usually <10mmHg.
b.   It usually signifies occlusion in a branch of the right coronary artery.
c.   Right to left shunting is a recognised complication.
d.   Inferior myocardial infarction is usually present.
e.   Right coronary artery occlusion is usually present.

A10   Which of the following is TRUE concerning vascular access devices?

a.   The flow of crystalloid through a 16G intravenous cannula is approximately 150ml/min.
b.   Laminar flow is proportional to the viscosity of the fluid.
c.   Laminar flow is proportional to the square of the radius.
d.   A central line is the most effective means of fluid resuscitation for a trauma patient.
e.   Intraosseous access is contraindicated in adult patients.

A11 Which of the following is NOT a component of the Lund protocol for the management of traumatic brain injury?

a. Routine use of antihypertensives including clonidine and metoprolol.
b. Transfusion of albumin to 40g/L.
c. Acceptance of a cerebral perfusion pressure of 50mmHg.
d. Use of dihydroergotamine to reduce cerebral venous blood volume.
e. Low-dose mannitol infusion.

A12 The following are prerequisites for the use of recombinant factor VIIa in bleeding trauma patients EXCEPT:

a. Platelet count >50x10^9/L.
b. Temperature >36°C.
c. Fibrinogen >0.5g/L.
d. pH >7.20.
e. Ionised Ca^{2+} >0.8mmol/L (3.2mg/dL).

A13 Which of the following statements regarding the use of antifibrinolytic agents is FALSE?

a. Tranexamic acid is a competitive inhibitor of plasminogen and plasmin.
b. Aprotinin significantly reduces blood loss and transfusion requirements in cardiac surgery.
c. Use of antifibrinolytics in trauma is supported by several high quality randomised controlled trials.
d. Arterial and venous thrombosis are uncommon complications of tranexamic acid use.
e. The risk of anaphylaxis with aprotinin is 0.5%.

A14 A 48-year-old woman is rescued from a house fire during which she was trapped in a smoke-filled bedroom for 30 minutes. On arrival in the Emergency Room, she has marked facial burns and a hoarse voice but no stridor. She is expectorating carbonaceous sputum, appears confused and has a cherry-red visage. Which statement is FALSE?

a. Early intubation is advisable.
b. A significant thermal injury to the trachea is likely.
c. Lavage with sodium bicarbonate 1.4% has a role in the management of this patient.
d. Lung function is likely to worsen over the next 12 hours.
e. A cherry red visage has several causes other than carbon monoxide poisoning.

A15 All the following increase the likelihood of a patient acquiring an antimicrobial-resistant infection EXCEPT:

a. Use of cefotaxime.
b. High nursing workload.
c. Prolonged mechanical ventilation.
d. Brief hospital admission.
e. Understaffing in the ICU.

A16 A 77-year-old man is admitted to the cardiac intensive care unit (ICU) following an elective triple vessel coronary artery bypass graft. On day 3 of his stay he is noted to be hypotensive and oliguric with a BP of 75/50mmHg and a HR of 125bpm (regular). Pulmonary artery catheter data show: pulmonary artery pressure 15/7mmHg, central venous pressure 3mmHg, pulmonary artery occlusion pressure 5mmHg, cardiac index 1.6L/min/m^2, systemic vascular resistance 2750 dyne/sec/cm^5. The MOST LIKELY diagnosis is:

a. Cardiac failure.
b. Cardiac tamponade.
c. Sepsis.
d. Hypovolaemia.
e. Pulmonary embolism.

A17 A 74-year-old lady with a history of ischaemic heart disease and severe congestive cardiac failure is admitted to the ICU with hypotension and presumed sepsis. She is sedated and ventilated in pressure support mode. On examination she is confused, BP is 85/35mmHg, HR is 115bpm (sinus tachycardia), SpO$_2$ is 95% on 60% oxygen. Arterial blood gas analysis shows a lactate of 4.3mmol/L (39mg/dL). Which is the BEST guide to the need for further intravenous fluid replacement?

a. Response of oesophageal Doppler to passive leg raising.
b. Insertion of a pulmonary artery catheter and pulmonary artery occlusion pressure measurement.
c. Titrate fluid resuscitation against repeated blood lactate measurements.
d. Assess pulse pressure variation.
e. Urine output measurement.

A18 Which one of the following statements is TRUE regarding physical methods of temperature measurement?

a. The lower limit for use of a mercury thermometer is 30.5°C.
b. The upper limit for use of an alcohol thermometer is 90°C.
c. A Bourdon gauge thermometer uses units of kPa or mmHg.
d. A bimetallic strip is typically composed of brass and stainless steel.
e. A constant volume gas thermometer is explained by Charles' law.

A19 The following are true regarding sources of error in pulse oximetry EXCEPT:

a. Use of local anaesthetic may cause a fall in SpO_2.
b. Jaundice does not affect the signal.
c. Severe tricuspid regurgitation reduces the SpO_2 reading.
d. Readings are unreliable below 70% SpO_2.
e. Foetal haemoglobin (HbF) causes overestimation of SpO_2.

A20 Which ONE of the following is the most useful indicator when considering a diagnosis of massive pulmonary embolism?

a. A fall in end-tidal CO_2 to 1.3kPa.
b. A pulmonary artery pressure of 22/10mmHg.
c. An oxygen saturation of 88% on room air.
d. An arterial blood gas showing a PaO_2 of 6.5kPa on room air.
e. S1Q3T3 pattern on the ECG.

A21 A 28-year-old man is transferred to the ICU following a road traffic accident for which he required a splenectomy, packing of a liver laceration and laparostomy. Thirty minutes after he has been established on mechanical ventilation the following capnograph trace is seen:

This trace is best explained by:

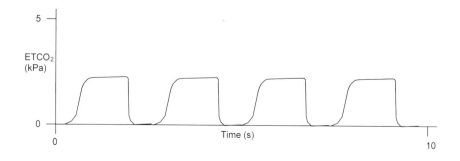

a. A fall in cardiac output.
b. Disconnection of the noradrenaline infusion.
c. Hyperventilation.
d. Fat embolism.
e. Bronchospasm.

A22 The following statements are true regarding daily interruption of sedation on the ICU EXCEPT:

a. Length of ICU stay is reduced.
b. The drug-sparing effect is greater with propofol than midazolam.
c. The period of mechanical ventilation is shorter.
d. Fewer CT brain scans are required.
e. In-hospital mortality is unaffected.

A23 Placement of a vena cava filter should be considered in the following cases EXCEPT:

a. A patient requiring urgent major vascular surgery who was diagnosed with a proximal deep vein thrombosis 1 week previously.
b. A patient with malignancy who develops a pulmonary embolism despite maximal therapeutic anticoagulation (international normalised ratio [INR] 3.5).
c. A patient with a recent intracerebral haemorrhage who develops a proximal deep vein thrombosis.
d. A pregnant patient who develops a pulmonary embolism 2 weeks before her expected date of delivery.
e. A patient newly diagnosed with the antiphospholipid syndrome.

A24 The following are true of the serotonin syndrome EXCEPT:

a. It may be precipitated by monoamine oxidase inhibitors.
b. Cyproheptadine is part of the treatment of the syndrome.
c. Extrapyramidal signs are not present.
d. Onset is rapid over a period of hours.
e. It is an idiosyncratic drug reaction.

A25 Which of the following is most strongly predictive of outcome in acute pancreatitis?

a.   Serum amylase.
b.   Serum lipase.
c.   C-reactive protein.
d.   Bilirubin.
e.   White cell count.

A26 The ECG shown below is consistent with:

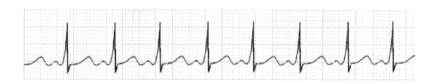

a.   Complete heart block.
b.   Sick sinus syndrome.
c.   Wolff-Parkinson-White syndrome.
d.   Brugada syndrome.
e.   Atrial fibrillation.

A27 An essential prerequisite of organ donation for transplantation is:

a.   Discussion with relatives about the deceased's wishes.
b.   Noradrenaline or dopamine infusion.
c.   Thyroid hormone supplementation.
d.   A cocktail of medications for cardiac donation.
e.   None of the above.

A28 A 63-year-old man with a history of idiopathic pulmonary fibrosis (IPF) is referred to the ICU with progressive dyspnoea and Type I respiratory failure. Which statement is TRUE?

a. Non-invasive ventilation is a useful therapeutic option.
b. Pneumonia is the commonest cause of worsening respiratory failure in patients with IPF.
c. The outlook is good for patients who survive their ICU admission.
d. An infectious cause of respiratory deterioration improves the prognosis.
e. FEV_1 is not a useful predictor of ICU survival.

A29 A 23-year-old asthmatic presents to the Emergency Room with dyspnoea and diffuse wheeze. He has a RR of 40 breaths per minute, a HR of 120bpm (sinus tachycardia) and an SpO_2 of 90% on 15L/min oxygen via a non-rebreathing mask. He is unable to talk in sentences but is fully alert and obviously frightened. He has had two nebulisers in the ambulance on the way to hospital with little improvement. The following are appropriate treatments EXCEPT:

a. Nebulised ipratropium bromide 0.5mg driven with oxygen.
b. Heliox.
c. Intravenous magnesium sulphate 2g.
d. Intravenous aminophylline 5mg/kg over 20 minutes.
e. Oral prednisolone 50mg.

A30 A 35-year-old polytrauma victim develops acute respiratory distress syndrome (ARDS) while ventilated on the ICU. Proning is considered. Which one of the following statements is TRUE?

a. There is level 1 evidence for a mortality benefit from proning in ARDS.
b. Proning may be of greater benefit in ARDS patients with higher PaO_2/FiO_2 ratios.
c. The optimum duration of proning is generally held to be 6 hours/day.
d. Proning may be of greater benefit in patients with higher severity of illness scores.
e. The is level 1 evidence to prove that proning does not improve outcome.

A31 A 76-year-old woman is seen in the Emergency Room with palpitations and shortness of breath. She is known to have atrial fibrillation for which she takes digoxin. On examination she has bibasal crackles on chest auscultation, a blood pressure of 80/50mmHg and an SpO$_2$ of 87% on 15L/min oxygen via a non-rebreathing mask. The ECG shows atrial fibrillation with a ventricular rate of 170bpm. Although she takes warfarin, her INR is 1.3 on laboratory testing. The most appropriate initial course of action is:

a. Rate control with intravenous digoxin and therapeutic anticoagulation.
b. Intravenous metoprolol for immediate rate control.
c. Valsalva manoeuvre.
d. Induction of anaesthesia and synchronised DC shock.
e. Intravenous amiodarone in view of the subtherapeutic anticoagulation.

A32 Regarding the use of the intra-aortic balloon pump (IABP) for cardiac failure, which one of the following statements is FALSE?

a. The IABP must be inserted via the femoral artery.
b. The balloon inflates immediately following the dicrotic notch on the arterial waveform.
c. The balloon deflates during isovolumetric contraction of the left ventricle.
d. The augmentation pressure is the peak pressure produced during IABP inflation in diastole.
e. Systolic blood pressure usually decreases during IABP use.

A33 Which of the following is the LEAST useful initial investigation in a systemically well patient presenting to the Emergency Room with a sudden onset hemianopia, right arm weakness and dysphasia?

a. Full blood count.
b. Chest X-ray.
c. Electrocardiogram.
d. Serum glucose.
e. CT brain scan.

A34 A 38-year-old lady presents with slurred speech, diplopia and respiratory insufficiency of recent onset. Examination is unremarkable apart from a small goitre. There is no history of autonomic disturbance. There is no history of foreign travel (she lives in the UK). She has no rashes and is not systemically unwell. No history of antecedent infection is noted. Which of the following is the most likely diagnosis?

a. Myasthenia gravis.
b. Botulism.
c. Lyme disease.
d. Charcot-Marie-Tooth disease.
e. Guillain-Barré syndrome.

A35 The following statements are true concerning the management of acute renal failure in the ICU with intermittent haemodialysis (IHD) or continuous renal replacement therapy (CRRT) EXCEPT:

a. The maximal safe rate of fluid removal with IHD is 250ml/h.
b. Clearance of urea (ml/min) is much greater with IHD than CRRT.
c. Mortality is similar in ICU patients treated with IHD or CRRT.
d. IHD can be used successfully in haemodynamically unstable patients.
e. CRRT is more labour-intensive for the ICU staff.

A36 A 54-year-old epileptic man is found on the floor in a post-ictal state at home. He is brought to the Emergency Room where he is noted to be oliguric on urinary catheterisation. Urine tests are positive for myoglobin. The following blood tests are typical of early rhabdomyolysis EXCEPT:

a.   Elevated serum creatinine.
b.   Hyperuricaemia.
c.   Hypercalcaemia.
d.   Hyperphosphataemia.
e.   Hyperkalaemia.

A37 A 48-year-old epileptic presents following ingestion of 30 500mg paracetamol tablets 6 hours ago. He states that he wishes to die. Which one of the following statements is TRUE?

a.   Serious liver damage is unlikely if N-acetylcysteine is given within 12 hours of ingestion.
b.   His epilepsy medication may provide some protection.
c.   N-acetylcysteine must not be continued for >24h.
d.   A pH of <7.3 on initial presentation is an indication for liver transplantation.
e.   A raised alanine aminotransferase (ALT) level is the most sensitive prognostic marker.

A38 A septic patient on the ICU is noted to be oozing blood from a central venous catheter insertion site. The following laboratory tests support a diagnosis of disseminated intravascular coagulation EXCEPT:

a.   Platelet count of 50×10^9/L.
b.   Prothrombin time of 52 seconds.
c.   Target cells on the blood film.
d.   Prolonged thrombin time.
e.   Fibrinogen 0.5g/L.

A39 A 55-year-old patient with known oesophageal varices has an upper gastro-intestinal bleed requiring a six-unit blood transfusion. He became encephalopathic and was intubated and is now ventilated on the ICU. He continues to bleed. The most appropriate therapy would be:

a. Somatostatin.
b. Propranolol.
c. Endoscopic variceal banding.
d. Conservative management and correction of coagulopathy.
e. Gastro-oesophageal balloon tamponade.

A40 The following radiological features are matched with the correct diagnosis EXCEPT:

a. Silhouette sign and pneumothorax.
b. Pleural capping and dissecting thoracic aorta.
c. Bat's wing shadowing and cardiogenic pulmonary oedema.
d. Air bronchogram and consolidation.
e. Wedge-shaped shadow and pulmonary embolism.

A41 Which of the following is NOT a complication of cocaine poisoning?

a. Impairment of haemostasis.
b. Ischaemic stroke.
c. Extrapyramidal movement disorders.
d. Pneumonitis.
e. Gastroduodenal perforation.

A42 Phencyclidine (PCP) is a recreational drug of abuse. It is a weak base (pKa 9) which is highly lipid-soluble and 78% protein-bound. It has cholinergic, anticholinergic, sympathomimetic, dopaminergic, narcotic and serotonergic effects. It is metabolised by the liver to inactive metabolites. 10% of the active drug is excreted in the urine. Based on this information the following are true EXCEPT:

a. Urinary acidification will enhance renal elimination of the drug.
b. Phencyclidine crosses the placenta.
c. Haemodialysis is likely to be an effective therapy for overdose.
d. Hypertension is likely.
e. Volume of distribution is likely to exceed 1L/kg.

A43 Regarding the circulatory physiology of pregnancy which statement is FALSE?

a. Systemic vascular resistance normally falls in early pregnancy.
b. The renin-angiotensin-aldosterone system is up-regulated.
c. Systolic pressure decreases to a lesser extent than diastolic.
d. Hypertension in pregnancy is essentially harmful only to the foetus.
e. Hypertension detected in the first trimester is likely to be longstanding.

A44 A 33-week pregnant patient with known pre-eclampsia is brought to the Emergency Room with an isolated head injury caused by a blow to the left temple. On examination her GCS is 6 and she has a fixed and dilated left pupil. Blood pressure is 170/115mmHg. She has no signs of extracranial injury, and the cardiotocograph shows no abnormality. Plans are made to intubate and ventilate the patient in order to facilitate an urgent CT brain scan. Which one of the following statements is TRUE?

a. The baby must be delivered by Caesarean section prior to a CT scan.
b. Opiates should be avoided during induction of anaesthesia.
c. Pre-eclampsia is a predictor of difficult laryngoscopy.
d. Sodium nitroprusside is the first-line agent for blood pressure control.
e. Intravenous lignocaine 1mg/kg should be given to attenuate the pressor response to intubation.

A45 The following are true of dobutamine administration EXCEPT:

a. Left ventricular end-diastolic pressure (LVEDP) is reduced.
b. It has a half-life of 2 minutes.
c. Systemic vascular resistance is reduced.
d. Cardiac index is increased.
e. It is contraindicated in patients with known ischaemic heart disease.

A46 A patient on the ICU is hypotensive for a period of days secondary to severe sepsis. Regarding the expected effect that this will have on the hepatic metabolism of drugs, which one of the following statements is FALSE?

a. Liver blood flow is likely to be greatly reduced in this patient.
b. Midazolam will accumulate significantly.
c. Remifentanil can be used as normal.
d. Hepatic metabolism of flow-limited drugs will be significantly impaired.
e. Hepatic metabolism of drugs with a low extraction ratio will be significantly impaired.

A47 A patient on the high dependency unit has pneumonia and is hypoxic on room air. When deciding which method of oxygen administration is appropriate which of the following statements is FALSE?

a. Maximum inspiratory flow may exceed 30L/min during spontaneous breathing.
b. Nasal cannulae significantly improve oxygenation even if the patient breathes through the mouth.
c. A Venturi mask uses the Bernoulli principle.
d. A Hudson mask is a fixed performance device.
e. An anaesthetic face mask increases dead space.

A48 A 75-year-old man develops a *Clostridium difficile* infection on the ICU following a course of ceftriaxone for community-acquired pneumonia (this antibiotic has now been stopped). He has a white cell count of 25×10^9/L and a serum creatinine of 230µmol/L (2.6mg/dL). The most appropriate initial treatment is:

a. Oral metronidazole.
b. Oral vancomycin.
c. Intravenous metronidazole.
d. Intravenous vancomycin.
e. Nasojejunal faecal replacement.

A49 Which of the following is the commonest adverse incident in the ICU?

a. Inappropriate alarm settings.
b. Line, drain and catheter dislodgement.
c. Airway obstruction/dislodgement.
d. Medication errors.
e. Equipment failure.

A50 A patient attends the ICU follow-up clinic 3 months after discharge following a prolonged period of several weeks' mechanical ventilation with abdominal sepsis, multiple organ failure and prolonged weaning from the ventilator. He did not receive a tracheostomy. He complains of shortness of breath on exertion and an inability to exhale effectively. Flow-volume loop studies show the following:

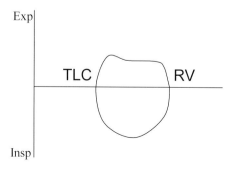

The most likely diagnosis is:

a.   Interstitial lung disease.
b.   Bronchospasm.
c.   Tracheal stenosis.
d.   Tracheomalacia.
e.   None of the above.

Paper 1

Type 'K' questions

K51 A 64-year-old man presents with a progressive history of nausea, lethargy, confusion and headache over several days. He has had a recent diagnosis of small cell bronchogenic carcinoma. He suffers a generalised seizure which spontaneously terminates. Initial blood tests show a plasma sodium of 115mmol/l. The following support a diagnosis of the syndrome of inappropriate antidiuretic hormone secretion (SIADH):

a. Urine sodium less than 20mmol/l.
b. Correction by water restriction.
c. Pitting oedema.
d. Urine osmolality greater than plasma osmolality.

K52 The following may be signs of hypomagnesaemia:

a. Trousseau's and Chvostek's signs.
b. Hyperreflexia.
c. Flushing.
d. Ataxia.

K53 Regarding microshock:

a. Risk of ventricular fibrillation is proportional to current density.
b. Microshock is unlikely with leakage currents at mains frequency (50Hz).
c. Microshock is unlikely with a leakage current of <50µA.
d. Type CF equipment is for cardiac use and has a floating circuit.

K54 Regarding the use of therapeutic hypothermia in cardiac arrest survivors:

a. Level 1 evidence exists in out-of-hospital cardiac arrest patients with return of spontaneous circulation.
b. Cooling should begin as soon as possible.
c. There is no significant difference in the incidence of arrhythmia compared with normothermic controls.
d. Therapeutic hypothermia should be continued for at least 72 hours once instituted.

K55 While crossing the road, a 55-year-old man is struck in the right side of the chest by the handlebar of a passing motorbike travelling at speed. On arrival in the Emergency Room his oxygenation deteriorates and he requires intubation and ventilation. A post-intubation chest X-ray shows fractures of right ribs 5-9 inclusive, with clear lung fields. No other injuries are identified on secondary survey. Arterial blood gas analysis shows: pH 7.23, PCO_2 8.5kPa (64mmHg), PO_2 9.6kPa (73mmHg), base excess -4.5mmol/L (FiO_2 0.8).

a. A chest drain should be inserted immediately.
b. A CT thorax may provide additional diagnostic information.
c. Steroids are not indicated.
d. Ventilation in the right lateral position is likely to improve oxygenation.

K56 A 41-year-old car driver hits a wall head-on at 50 miles per hour. She is quickly extricated and brought to the Emergency Room complaining of abdominal pain. No extra-abdominal injuries are identified on initial assessment. Seatbelt marks are visible on the abdomen. Blood tests include a haemoglobin concentration of 11.5g/dL, amylase of 60IU/L, and aspartate aminotransferase (AST) of 500IU/L.

a. Mesenteric injury is a significant concern.
b. Pancreatic injury is excluded by a normal amylase.
c. The raised AST should increase suspicion of hepatic injury.
d. Hypotensive resuscitation should be employed.

K57 A 19-year-old male is thrown from a motorbike in a road traffic accident. On arrival in the Emergency Room he is treated with fluids and oxygen, and is haemodynamically stable with no obvious truncal or limb injuries. Prior to rapid sequence induction of anaesthesia he has a GCS of 5 with extensor posturing, and dilated fixed pupils. A CT brain scan shows a 6mm midline shift and diffuse petechial haemorrhages.

a.   The GCS post-resuscitation has prognostic significance.
b.   Midline shift of >5mm on the CT scan carries a poor prognosis.
c.   A 48-hour infusion of intravenous methylprednisolone is indicated.
d.   The verbal response is the most prognostically useful component of the GCS.

K58 The following findings in cerebrospinal fluid are characteristic of the Guillain-Barré syndrome:

a.   Pleocytosis.
b.   CSF glucose >2/3 of plasma glucose.
c.   Protein >0.5g/L.
d.   Oligoclonal bands.

K59 A 78-year-old man presents with a seizure 5 days post-carotid endarterectomy. It spontaneously terminates but on recovery he complains of a severe left-sided 'pounding' headache and a weak right arm. His BP is 205/110mmHg.

a.   A CT brain scan is not required.
b.   His blood pressure should be reduced by pharmacological means.
c.   Glyceryl trinitrate is the agent of choice.
d.   A heparin infusion should be started immediately.

K60 Regarding sites of vascular access:

a.   The brachial artery lies between the biceps brachii tendon and the ulnar nerve.
b.   The femoral nerve travels in the femoral canal with the femoral vein and artery.
c.   The carotid sheath contains the internal jugular vein, carotid artery and vagus nerve.
d.   The long saphenous vein can be cannulated 2cm posterior and superior to the medial malleolus.

K61 Regarding the intensive care management of patients with blunt traumatic brain injury:

a.   Hyperglycaemia has no bearing on neurological outcome.
b.   The incidence of deep vein thrombosis is less than 10% in isolated head injury.
c.   Prophylactic anticoagulation for thromboprophylaxis should begin in the first 24h.
d.   Prophylactic hypothermia is a standard of care in the management of these patients.

K62 A 48-year-old man falls five stories from a window suffering significant abdominal injuries. During laparotomy liver lacerations and diffuse small vessel bleeding are identified. The abdomen is packed and the patient is transferred to the ICU. Over the next 6 hours he continues to bleed requiring a six-unit blood transfusion. A haematology opinion is sought regarding the use of recombinant factor VIIa (rFVIIa).

a.   rFVIIa is not licensed for use in this situation.
b.   rFVIIa has been shown to reduce blood transfusion requirements in blunt trauma.
c.   Use of rFVIIa is proven to reduce mortality in blunt trauma.
d.   The action of rFVIIa is independent of platelet number and function.

K63 A 44-year-old man is involved in a road traffic accident and is admitted to the ICU following fluid and blood resuscitation, emergency splenectomy, external fixation of a pelvic fracture and external fixation of a femoral shaft fracture. On initial presentation in the Emergency Room he was in ATLS grade III shock and arterial blood gas analysis showed a lactate of 6.4mmol/L (58mg/dL); on arrival in the ICU this has reduced to 3.5mmol/L (32mg/dL).

a.   This man has a Type A lactic acidosis.
b.   Lactate is of prognostic significance in trauma patients.
c.   Venous blood can be used for lactate analysis.
d.   Outlook will be poor if lactate remains above 2mmol/L after 48h.

K64 A 30-year-old woman presents to the Emergency Room following a suicide attempt where she has been in an enclosed space with a burning coal fire. She is drowsy (GCS 13) with a HR of 123bpm, a BP of 125/95mmHg, and oxygen saturation of 96% on high-flow oxygen. She has a brief tonic-clonic seizure which self-terminates. Arterial blood gas analysis shows: pH 7.36, PO_2 40.6kPa (308mmHg), PCO_2 4.4kPa (33mmHg), calculated SaO_2 99%.

a.   The history and findings are consistent with carbon monoxide poisoning.
b.   There is evidence of a saturation gap.
c.   Oxygen therapy should be titrated down to a lower PaO_2.
d.   Hyperbaric oxygen therapy is contraindicated.

K65 Concerning the measurement of cardiac output by thermodilution techniques:

a.   A pulmonary artery catheter is required.
b.   Cardiac output is inversely proportional to the area under the temperature-time curve.
c.   A small volume of injectate will underestimate cardiac output.
d.   'Cold' injectate should be at 12-15°C.

K66 The following assumptions are made when determining stroke volume using an oesophageal Doppler probe:

a. 70% of total cardiac output passes the probe.
b. The ascending aorta runs parallel to the oesophagus.
c. The diameter of the aorta is constant throughout systole.
d. Haematocrit is unchanged between measurements.

K67 Regarding the management of carbon monoxide poisoning:

a. The half-life of carboxyhaemoglobin in air is about 4 hours.
b. A carboxyhaemoglobin level of 60% is commonly lethal.
c. An otherwise fit and well patient with a carboxyhaemoglobin level of 50% will have an arterial oxygen content of approximately $5mlO_2/100ml$ when breathing 100% oxygen.
d. Untreated pneumothorax is an absolute contraindication to hyperbaric oxygen therapy.

K68 The following information can be derived from the arterial pressure waveform:

a. Stroke volume from the area under the entire waveform.
b. Myocardial afterload from dP/dt.
c. Hypovolaemia from a high dicrotic notch.
d. Vasodilatation from a steep diastolic rate of decay.

K69 Regarding the physical principles behind pulse oximetry:

a. Light is transmitted through the measurement site at 3Hz.
b. Light is transmitted at wavelengths of 660nm (red) and 940nm (infrared).
c. The isobestic point indicates an SpO_2 of 50%.
d. The Hagen-Poiseuille law underpins the physics involved.

K70 A 43-year-old woman presents with shortness of breath, pleuritic chest pain and haemoptysis. Oxygen saturation is 87% on air, RR is 45 breaths per minute, HR is 156bpm, BP is 80/55mmHg. The echocardiogram shows moderate right ventricular dilatation with an estimated pulmonary artery pressure of 60mmHg.

a. Pulmonary embolism is a likely diagnosis.
b. The mortality rate is around 1% with this clinical picture.
c. Thrombolysis has been shown to reduce the risk of death for such patients.
d. A left ventricular heave is a likely finding on examination.

K71 The capnograph trace below could be explained by:

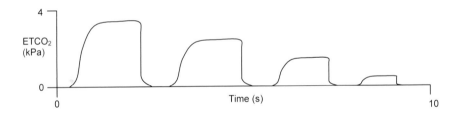

a. Oesophageal intubation.
b. Endobronchial intubation.
c. Massive haemorrhage.
d. Hyperventilation.

K72 Regarding the following intracranial pressure trace:

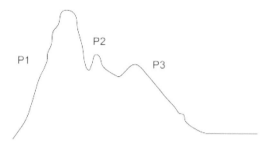

a. P1 represents transmitted arterial pulsation.
b. P2 exceeds P1 as intracranial compliance falls.
c. P3 represents the dicrotic notch.
d. P1, P2 and P3 are Lundberg waves.

K73 Regarding the aetiology of massive haemoptysis:

a. It more commonly originates from the bronchial than the pulmonary circulation.
b. Chest X-ray identifies the source of bleeding in a minority of cases.
c. The presence of a nasal septal perforation may suggest Behcet's syndrome.
d. Pulmonary-renal syndromes are the commonest cause.

K74 The following blood tests are available from a patient just admitted to the ICU: sodium 145mmol/L, potassium 3.5mmol/L, urea 17mmol/L (BUN 48mg/dL), creatinine 170μmol/L (1.9mg/dL), bicarbonate 8mmol/L, chloride 105mmol/L, glucose 30mmol/L (550mg/dL). Regarding this patient:

a. The anion gap is raised.
b. The serum osmolality is raised.
c. The biochemical picture is consistent with gastric outflow obstruction.
d. Excessive administration of 0.9% saline can cause this biochemical picture.

K75 Concerning aortic dissection:

a.   Medical management is the preferred option in uncomplicated Stanford Type B dissection.
b.   Medical management includes noradrenaline infusion to maintain renal perfusion pressure.
c.   The commonest site of origin is the descending aorta.
d.   A transoesophageal echocardiogram is the investigation of choice in patients too unstable for angiography.

K76 Regarding the Injury Severity Score (ISS):

a.   It is comprised of anatomical and physiological data.
b.   The maximum score is 75.
c.   Head injury carries the highest weighting.
d.   Six body regions are defined.

K77 The following are good predictors of increased hospital mortality in patients with chronic obstructive pulmonary disease (COPD) requiring mechanical ventilation:

a.   Mechanical ventilation lasting >72h.
b.   An FEV_1 <30% predicted prior to ICU admission.
c.   One failed extubation attempt.
d.   Presence of comorbidities.

K78 Regarding therapeutic interventions for massive haemoptysis:

a.   Bronchial artery embolisation is successful in the majority of cases.
b.   Emergency lung resection carries a 60% mortality.
c.   Bronchoscopic lavage with epinephrine 1:10000 may be useful.
d.   Rigid bronchoscopy has no place in this situation.

K79 Regarding the use of positive end-expiratory pressure (PEEP) in patients with acute respiratory distress syndrome (ARDS):

a.   High PEEP (>12cmH$_2$O) reduces ICU mortality compared with low PEEP (5-12cmH$_2$O).
b.   PEEP should be set below the lower inflection point on the pressure-volume curve.
c.   High PEEP improves the PaO$_2$/FiO$_2$ ratio compared with low PEEP.
d.   PEEP causes atelectrauma.

K80 Regarding atrial fibrillation:

a.   Maximum cardiac output occurs with ventricular rate controlled to 50bpm.
b.   The atria are normally responsible for 40-50% of ventricular filling.
c.   Valvular heart disease is the commonest cause.
d.   'Atrial stunning' commonly occurs after successful cardioversion.

K81 The following are absolute contraindications to the use of an intra-aortic balloon pump:

a.   Clinically significant aortic stenosis.
b.   Refractory angina.
c.   Aortic dissection.
d.   Severe peripheral vascular disease.

K82 A 77-year-old man on the high dependency unit is found to have a new right-sided homonymous hemianopia and dysphasia on the afternoon ward round. His observations include: HR of 85bpm, BP of 190/105mmHg, SpO$_2$ of 96% on room air. A CT brain scan is unremarkable. Appropriate initial management includes:

a.   Aspirin 300mg.
b.   Clopidogrel 300mg.
c.   Treatment dose of low-molecular-weight heparin.
d.   Labetalol.

K83 The following features favour a diagnosis of encephalopathy over encephalitis in a patient presenting with an altered sensorium:

a. Meningism.
b. Normal cerebrospinal fluid analysis.
c. Gradual steady deterioration in mental status.
d. Seizures.

K84 The following interventions are effective in reducing the incidence of acute renal failure in selected populations:

a. Low dose dopamine infusion (2μg/kg/min).
b. Mannitol.
c. Normal saline infusion prior to administration of radiocontrast media.
d. N-acetylcysteine prior to administration of radiocontrast media.

K85 A 28-year-old intravenous drug-using woman is admitted to the ICU. She has been complaining of being itchy, and feeling lethargic and unwell. She is sleepy but rousable, and is incoherent and extremely confused. Asterixis is present. Serology confirms acute hepatitis B infection; the prothrombin time is 70 seconds.

a. This patient has grade III hepatic encephalopathy.
b. The clotting deficit should be corrected with fresh frozen plasma.
c. Survival rates for this condition without liver transplantation are around 60%.
d. Cerebral oedema is a likely cause of the confusional state.

K86 Regarding acalculous cholecystitis in the ICU patient:

a. It has a high mortality.
b. The incidence is around 0.2%.
c. Gram negative biliary tract sepsis is the initiating cause.
d. Ultrasonography is highly sensitive and specific for the condition.

K87 A 45-year-old man is admitted to the ICU with signs of sepsis. He complains of a painful, swollen knee for the last 3 days. There is no history of trauma and he has no previous history of joint problems or other medical problems. He is apyrexial, but has an erythrocyte sedimentation rate (ESR) of 72mm/h. A diagnosis of septic arthritis is considered.

a. Septic arthritis is unlikely in the absence of pyrexia.
b. An elevated ESR is a sensitive indicator of septic arthritis.
c. Plain radiography is often diagnostic.
d. A negative Gram stain of joint fluid aspirate excludes the diagnosis.

K88 Regarding the RIFLE criteria classification system for acute renal failure:

a. The 'E' in 'RIFLE' represents end-stage kidney disease.
b. Kidney failure can be diagnosed based on urine output alone.
c. Criteria for risk of kidney injury are specific but not sensitive.
d. Serum creatinine is accepted as an index of glomerular function.

K89 The following drugs require altered dosing in patients with advanced liver cirrhosis:

a. Midazolam.
b. Remifentanil.
c. Atracurium.
d. Propofol.

K90 When commencing renal replacement therapy, the following properties predict significantly increased clearance of a drug compared with the anuric state:

a. Low protein-binding.
b. Low volume of distribution.
c. High non-renal clearance.
d. High molecular weight.

K91 The following are common features of 3,4-methylene-dioxymethamphetamine ('ecstasy') poisoning:

a. Rhabdomyolysis.
b. Hypernatraemia.
c. Hyperthermia.
d. Non-cardiogenic pulmonary oedema.

K92 Regarding obstetric-related deaths in the developed world:

a. More mothers die from indirect causes (pre-existing disease exacerbated by pregnancy) than direct causes (bleeding, pre-eclampsia, etc.).
b. Haemorrhage is the leading direct cause of obstetric death.
c. Inability to intubate the patient is the leading cause of anaesthetic-related deaths.
d. Psychiatric disease is the commonest indirect cause of death.

K93 A patient with severe pre-eclampsia becomes unwell in the peripartum period with blurred vision, clonus and a BP of 180/120mmHg. The following are appropriate initial antihypertensive treatments:

a. Labetalol.
b. Hydralazine.
c. Nitroprusside.
d. Metolazone.

K94 A previously fit pregnant woman becomes mildly unwell in the third trimester and is admitted for routine investigations. On examination she has palmar erythema and several spider naevi. Liver function tests include: alkaline phosphatase 100IU/L, albumin 35g/L and alanine aminotransferase 35IU/L.

a.   Obstructive jaundice is likely to be present.
b.   There is evidence of pre-existing liver disease.
c.   Albumin is normally low in pregnancy (compared with non-pregnant values).
d.   Aminotransferases are normally elevated in the third trimester.

K95 Regarding noradrenaline (norepinephrine):

a.   A typical dose range would be 5-10µg/kg/min.
b.   It is a metabolite of adrenaline (epinephrine).
c.   It causes coronary artery vasodilatation increasing coronary blood flow.
d.   It increases contractility of the pregnant uterus.

K96 A postoperative patient on the high dependency unit has a morphine infusion running at 2mg/hour. The patient is still in pain following surgery, and the nursing staff ask you to adjust the morphine regime.

a.   Doubling the rate to 4mg/h will take about half an hour to have significant effect.
b.   The half-life of morphine is around 2-3 hours.
c.   If the clearance of morphine is halved by renal impairment, its half-life will double.
d.   The volume of distribution of morphine is around 0.5L/kg.

K97 The following data can be obtained from transpulmonary thermodilution:

a. Cardiac output.
b. An estimate of preload.
c. An estimate of pulmonary oedema.
d. An estimate of total circulating blood volume.

K98 Regarding pressure ulcers in the ICU:

a. A high Waterlow score is associated with an increased risk of pressure ulcer development.
b. Nursing workload increases by 50% if a pressure ulcer is present.
c. Pressure ulcers bear little relation to in-hospital mortality.
d. Patients with a pressure ulcer should be repositioned every 8 hours.

K99 Regarding the management of risk in the ICU and the techniques available for analysing risk factors:

a. The vast majority of clinical adverse incidents are due to a lack of technical skills in the medical staff.
b. Root cause analysis should be applied to all minor incidents in order to prevent future major incidents.
c. Observational studies using simulated patients are useful for assessing non-technical skills.
d. Attitudinal studies may not accurately reflect real life performance.

K100 Regarding tracheal stenosis as a complication of tracheostomy:

a. It most commonly occurs at the site of the tracheostomy tube cuff.
b. It is a much more common complication than tracheomalacia.
c. Patients rarely show symptoms in the first 3 months following decannulation.
d. Stridor is an early sign.

Paper 1

Type 'A' answers

A1   C

The maximum rate of potassium infusion should not exceed 40mmol/h as this may cause arrhythmias and asystole. Normal sodium requirement is 1-2mmol/day. Extracellular calcium exists in three forms: 40% protein bound (largely to albumin), 47% free ionised, and 13% complexed with citrate, phosphate and sulphate. The ionised form is the physiologically important one and may be reduced by alkalosis through greater protein binding. D and E are true as stated.

1.   Bersten AD, Soni N. *Oh's Intensive Care Manual,* 5th Ed. Edinburgh: Butterworth-Heinemann, 2003.

A2   B

This ECG shows a prolonged QT interval. This is defined as the distance between the beginning of the QRS complex and the end of the T wave. The QT interval in the ECG is around 14 small squares or 0.56 seconds (assuming a paper speed of 25mm/sec). Normal is 0.38-0.46s (9-11 small squares). The corrected QT interval (QTc) is given by Bazett's formula, QTc = QT/√R-R, adjusting for heart rate. Other causes of a long QT interval include electrolyte disturbances (hypokalaemia, hypomagnesaemia), congenital syndromes (Jervell-Lange-Neilsen, Romano-Ward) and drugs (antiarrhythmics, antimalarials, antihistamines and organophosphates).

1.   Ramrakha P, Moore K. *Oxford Handbook of Acute Medicine.* Oxford: Oxford University Press, 1997.

A3   D

A mains transformer isolates the power supply from earth. If a patient comes into contact with faulty equipment the current cannot flow through the patient to earth. An earth leakage circuit breaker switches off the electrical supply if stray currents are detected flowing to earth, reducing the potential for microshock. A common earth connects all the earthing points in a patient care area together reducing potential for microshock from earthing points at different potentials. Class II equipment has double insulation ensuring that even with one fault no part of the casing accessible to the patient is live. If the patient is earthed and comes into contact with faulty live equipment, the current will be conducted through the patient to earth causing burns.

1.   Davis PD, Parbrook GD, Kenny GN. *Basic Physics and Measurement in Anaesthesia,* 4th Ed. Oxford: Butterworth Heinemann, 2002.

A4   A

Iced water bodily immersion causes rapid cooling (9.7°C/h) but is impractical for routine use. Extracorporeal systems such as cardiac bypass are efficient but also impractical outside specialised units. Central venous cooling catheters are similar in size to a dialysis catheter but circulate cold fluid through a closed circuit and are effective cooling devices. Rapid infusion of large volumes of cold (4°C) crystalloid have been shown to effect cooling at a rate of 1.6°C/h and may also have beneficial effects by increasing cardiac output and mean arterial pressure. The use of cold air blankets, bladder irrigation and gastric lavage are all inefficient methods of cooling.

1.   Bernard SA, Buist M. Induced hypothermia in critical care medicine: a review. *Crit Care Med* 2003; 31(7): 2041-51.

A5   B

Traumatic cardiac tamponade is rare but should be suspected in the presence of sternal fracture, ECG changes and haemodynamic compromise. Beck's triad of elevated jugular venous pressure (JVP), muffled heart sounds and hypotension should be sought, although the first two features may be difficult to detect in the emergency setting. A widened cardiac shadow is not a sensitive sign for acute traumatic tamponade since only small volumes of blood (<500ml) in the pericardial space are required to cause haemodynamic compromise. Splenic rupture and pulmonary contusion are both possible diagnoses but should show some response to fluid therapy.

1. Ho AM. Cardiac tamponade and sternal fracture. *J Trauma* 2004; 56: 212-3.

A6   A

The use of albumin solutions in the initial resuscitation of trauma patients has not been shown to be more effective than the use of crystalloids. Blood substitutes such as polymerized haemoglobin are currently neither proven to be effective nor widely available. A prospective trial of field casualties with penetrating trauma randomised to immediate or delayed fluid resuscitation found better survival rates in the delayed fluid group (70% vs. 62% survival to hospital discharge) [1]. However, there is no evidence base for the use of this strategy in the hospital setting where immediate access to surgical haemorrhage control is available, and such a strategy may have deleterious effects on organ perfusion. A transfusion trigger of 7-9g/dL has been shown to be at least as safe as a higher threshold (10-12g/dL) in a large prospective study [2]; however, such triggers cannot be applied to the actively bleeding patient where fluid including blood products must be titrated against indicators of shock and end-organ perfusion.

1. Bickell WH, *et al.* Immediate versus delayed fluid resuscitation for hypotensive patients with penetrating torso injuries. *N Engl J Med* 1994; 331: 1105-9.
2. Hebert PC, *et al.* A multicenter, randomized, controlled clinical trial of transfusion requirements in critical care. *N Engl J Med* 1999; 340: 409-17.

A7   A

The recent MRC CRASH (Corticosteroid Randomisation After Significant Head Injury) trial data were used to determine a prognostic model for outcome (death at 14 days/disability at 6 months) based on data from 10,000 patients. Increasing age has a linear relationship with death over the age of 40. The risk of death also increases linearly with every point decrease in GCS. Dilated pupils and CT pathology including petechial haemorrhages, subarachnoid blood, midline shift and obliteration of the basal cisterns also increase the risk of death. Patient sex is not useful as a prognostic indicator. Using the CRASH head injury prognosis calculator this lady has a 14-day risk of death of 21% and a 6-month risk of death or severe disability of 71%.

1.   MRC CRASH Trial Collaborators. Predicting outcome after traumatic brain injury: practical prognostic models based on large cohort of international patients. *BMJ* 2008; 336: 425-9.

A8   A

Tuberculous meningitis occurs in immigrants, the homeless, alcoholics and, increasingly, in HIV positive patients. Caseous microtubercles develop in the brain and meninges; rupture causes infection and irritation of the meninges. Hydrocephalus is common, usually communicating and due to obliteration of the basal cisterns. A non-specific prodromal illness lasting several weeks is common. Examination findings include papilloedema in 40%, and cranial nerve palsies (most commonly VI). Arteritis may cause cerebral infarction. Lumbar puncture shows low glucose, moderately elevated protein, and classically a lymphocytic pleocytosis (although a CSF neutrophilia is common in the early stages, and an acellular picture may be found in HIV-related cases). A Ziehl-Nielsen stain may show tubercles, culture will be positive in 50-80% of cases, and the polymerase chain reaction is a sensitive test. A positive India ink stain suggests cryptococcus, although a negative stain does not rule this out. The low glucose is against a diagnosis of viral meningitis, while the long prodrome and lymphocytic picture are against pneumococcal meningitis.

1.   Warrell DA, Farrar JJ, Crook DWM. Infections of the nervous system. In: *Oxford Textbook of Medicine*, 3rd Ed. Oxford: Oxford University Press, 2004.

A9   A

Right atrial pressure is usually elevated and greater than 10mmHg. Right ventricular infarction rarely occurs in isolation and is usually accompanied by inferior infarction. The posterior descending branch of the right coronary artery supplies the inferior and posterior walls of the right ventricle. Right to left shunting can occur at the atrial level through a patent foramen ovale in the presence of elevated right atrial pressure and should be suspected in patients who are hypoxic despite 100% oxygen (anatomical shunt).

1. Liu   RC.   Right   ventricular   infarction.   Available: http://www.emedicine.com/MED/topic2039.htm. Last accessed 20 November 2008.

A10   A

The Hagen-Poiseuille law states that flow is proportional to the fourth power of the radius, and to the pressure gradient, and is inversely proportional to the viscosity of the fluid and the length of the tube. Hence, a central line is a less efficient means of delivering fluid than a standard intravenous cannula of the same gauge. Intraosseous access is permissible in adults if intravenous access is not possible, though the tougher bony cortex makes this difficult. The tibia, sternum and iliac crest are all potential sites.

1. Kenny G, Davis P. *Basic Physics and Measurement in Anaesthesia*, 5th Ed. Oxford: Butterworth-Heinemann, 2003.

A11   E

Traditional teaching emphasises the importance of maintaining a cerebral perfusion pressure (CPP) adequate to prevent brain ischaemia in the presence of a raised intracranial pressure (ICP). The Lund protocol focuses on the importance of Starling's forces in the development of brain oedema in the presence of disordered cerebral autoregulation following traumatic brain injury. Hence, blood pressure is limited to pre-injury normal levels (to prevent increased pre-capillary pressure in the presence of impaired arteriolar autoregulation) using metoprolol and clonidine. Albumin is transfused to maintain plasma colloid oncotic pressure. Thiopentone is used to promote arteriolar vasoconstriction (secondary to flow-metabolism coupling), and dihydroergotamine is used to promote venoconstriction and reduce cerebral blood volume. A minimum CPP of 50mmHg is accepted to minimise administration of inotropes and vasopressors which might increase cerebral oedema by increasing cerebral blood volume.

1.   Eker C, *et al.* Improved outcome after severe head injury with a new therapy based on principles for brain volume regulation and preserved microcirculation. *Crit Care Med* 1998; 26(11): 1881-6.

A12   B

Recombinant factor VIIa (rFVIIa) may be helpful to induce coagulation in areas of diffuse small vessel coagulopathic bleeding. It follows that all surgical avenues to control bleeding must first be explored. Adequate platelet numbers are required to generate the 'thrombin burst' which the rFVIIa provokes, and adequate fibrinogen must be present to translate this thrombin generation into clot formation. Correction of severe acidosis, hypothermia and hypocalcaemia are also warranted to maximise the chances of success for this expensive and unlicensed therapy. However, a temperature of 36°C is difficult to achieve in such patients; 32°C is considered an appropriate minimum threshold.

1.   Spahn DR, *et al.* Management of bleeding following major trauma: a European guideline. *Crit Care* 2007; 11(1): R17.

A13   C

Tranexamic acid (TXA) is a competitive inhibitor of plasmin and plasminogen, while aprotinin forms irreversible complexes with a variety of proteases including plasmin. While TXA is synthetic, aprotinin is isolated from bovine lungs and has a high incidence of anaphylaxis (0.5%). A strong evidence base supports the use of antifibrinolytic agents in cardiac surgery, where they have been shown to reduce the requirement for blood transfusion by about 30%. A Cochrane review [1] failed to demonstrate any increased incidence of thrombosis with antifibrinolytics, although a recent study [2] suggested that aprotinin is associated with an increased incidence of myocardial infarction, stroke and renal failure, leading to its withdrawal in the USA. The rationale for use in trauma is extrapolated from evidence in elective cardiac surgery; the ongoing CRASH (Clinical Randomisation of an Antifibrinolytic in Significant Haemorrhage) II trial should help determine whether they are effective in this context.

1. Hendy DA, *et al.* Anti-fibrinolytic use for minimising perioperative allogeneic blood transfusion. *Cochrane Database Syst Rev* 2001; (1): CD001886
2. Mangano DT, Tudor IC, Dietzel C. The risk associated with aprotinin in cardiac surgery. *New Engl J Med* 2006; 354: 353-65.

A14   B

Inhalational injury has three mechanisms: thermal injury to the upper airway, smoke inhalation causing chemical pneumonitis to the lower airways, and systemic absorption of toxins (principally carbon monoxide and cyanide). Hoarseness and facial burns are signs of upper airway thermal injury to the pharynx and glottic area. Pharyngeal oedema is likely to increase rapidly especially once fluid resuscitation is commenced, and early intubation is advised. Most of the heat from hot gas inhalation is dissipated in the upper airways, so thermal injury below the glottis is unusual. Sodium bicarbonate lavage of the bronchial tree may be performed following intubation to neutralise acidic deposits and remove soot contamination, although evidence for the effectiveness of this therapy is lacking. Lung function usually worsens over a period of hours following inhalational injury. A cherry red visage is a non-specific sign of carbon monoxide poisoning, and there are many other causes of facial flushing including alcohol, emotion and heat, all of which are associated with burns injuries.

1. Hilton PJ, Hepp M. The immediate care of the burned patient. *Continuing Education in Anaesthesia, Critical Care and Pain* 2001; 1(4): 113-6.

A15 D

Multi-drug resistant infections are increasing in incidence in the intensive care unit. Use of broad spectrum antibiotics such as third generation cephalosporins, carbapenems and quinolones is an independent risk factor for ventilator-acquired pneumonia with a drug-resistant organism, as is prolonged mechanical ventilation. Methycillin-resistant *Staphylococcus aureus* rates have been shown to increase with both overcrowding and understaffing of the ICU. Prolonged hospital admission, the presence of indwelling devices and poor hand hygiene also contribute to the development of antibiotic-resistant infections.

1. Salgado CD, O'Grady N, Farr BM. Prevention and control of antimicrobial-resistant infections in intensive care patients. *Crit Care Med* 2005; 33(10): 2373-82.

A16 D

All are clinically plausible diagnoses following cardiac surgery. However, the pulmonary artery catheter data are consistent with hypovolaemia. This may be due to drain losses, lack of intravenous fluids, GI tract losses, etc. Cardiac failure would be associated with high filling pressures, while tamponade would cause left and right ventricular diastolic pressures to equilibrate. Sepsis would be characterised by a high cardiac index (unless significant cardiac failure is present which is unlikely given the low filling pressures) and low systemic vascular resistance. Pulmonary embolism would be suggested by high pulmonary artery pressures and a high gradient between pulmonary artery diastolic pressure and pulmonary artery occlusion pressure.

1. Bowyer MW. Invasive haemodynamic monitoring. In: *Critical Care Secrets*, 3rd Ed. Parsons PE, Wiener-Kronish JP, Eds. London: Elsevier Health Sciences, 2003.

A17 A

This patient may have hypotension secondary to a variety of causes, including sepsis and decompensated cardiac failure. Pulmonary artery occlusion pressure has been shown to be a poor predictor of whether a fluid bolus will cause an increase in cardiac output (i.e. whether the patient is volume-responsive). Blood lactate is a sensitive marker of shock and falling levels correlate with improved survival. However, this will not distinguish between cardiogenic shock (where inotropes may be required) and septic shock (requiring fluids and/or vasopressors). Pulse pressure variation of >13% has been shown to accurately predict response to fluid, but is only reliable in mechanically ventilated patients without spontaneous respiratory effort. Urine output measurement will again not distinguish between different causes of shock. Passive leg raising autotransfuses about 300ml of blood into the central circulation. If stroke volume increases significantly (>10% as measured by oesophageal Doppler), this indicates preload-responsiveness. An advantage of this technique is that it is reversible if no improvement is seen, avoiding worsening pulmonary oedema in the case of cardiogenic shock.

1.   Antonelli M, *et al.* Haemodynamic monitoring in shock and implications for management. *Intensive Care Med* 2007; 33: 575-90.

A18   D

A mercury thermometer can be used to measure temperatures between -10 and 350°C. An alcohol thermometer can be used from -100 to 50°C. A Bourdon gauge thermometer (or any form of thermometer) uses units of temperature, not pressure! A bimetallic strip is typically made from brass and stainless steel, but could be composed of any two metals with different coefficients of thermal expansion. A constant volume gas thermometer exhibits a change in pressure which varies with temperature, assuming the gas is kept at a constant volume. The relationship between pressure and temperature is described by the third gas law (Gay-Lussac's law). Charles' law relates volume of a gas to temperature at constant pressure.

1.   Stoker MR. Measuring temperature. *Anaesthesia and Intensive Care Medicine* 2005; 6(6): 194-8.

A19 E

Prilocaine is a cause of methaemoglobinaemia, which tends to cause the SpO_2 to read around 85%. Jaundice, foetal haemoglobin and dark skin do not affect the accuracy of the measurement. The pulse oximeter estimates SpO_2 from the pulsatile component of the measured absorption spectrum (discarding the non-pulsatile venous and tissue component). Severe tricuspid regurgitation causes venous pulsation in the tissues (especially with ear probes), which causes deoxygenated but pulsatile venous blood to be measured, falsely lowering SpO_2. Readings below 70% are extrapolated rather than from direct reference data, and are therefore unreliable. However, any reading below 90% indicates serious hypoxaemia due to the steep fall in the oxygen dissociation curve at this point.

1.   Fearnley SJ. Pulse oximetry. *Update in Anaesthesia* 1995; Article 2.

A20 A

End tidal (ET) capnography in a ventilated patient usually reflects arterial $PaCO_2$, although $ETCO_2$ will always be around 0.5kPa less than $PaCO_2$ (in normal healthy lungs) due to a degree of V/Q mismatch. In a large pulmonary embolism, there is increased dead space (i.e. lung that is ventilated but not perfused) which will cause a large gap between alveolar (end tidal) and arterial CO_2; this is due to a fall in pulmonary blood flow. B is a normal pulmonary artery pressure; this may be raised in a large pulmonary embolism. C and D both reflect hypoxia, but do not indicate a cause. The classic $S_1Q_3T_3$ pattern is infrequently seen in cases of pulmonary embolism and is therefore insensitive.

1.   Bhavani Shankar K. (2001). Physiology of capnography. Available: http://www.capnography.com/Physiology/a-epd.htm. Last accessed 20 November 2008.

A21 C

The respiratory rate has been set at an inappropriately high level (around 24 breaths per minute) which will cause hypocapnia assuming that a normal tidal volume has been set (the end-tidal CO_2 is around 2.5kPa in the example given). If a fall in end-tidal CO_2 ($ETCO_2$) occurs rapidly in the presence of a normal minute volume, then both a fall in cardiac output and a hypotensive episode (including disconnection of vasopressors) must be considered. Pulmonary emboli may also cause a sudden fall in $ETCO_2$ as a result of increased physiological dead space, although this is more typical with air emboli or a massive pulmonary embolism than a fat embolus. Bronchospasm causes a slow rise in phases II and III of the capnograph trace with a characteristic sloping waveform (shown next to a normal trace below). A normal capnogram consists of four phases. Phase I represents the start of expiration, with dead space gas being expired. Phase II represents a mixture of dead space and alveolar gas being expired with progressive increase in partial pressure of CO_2. Phase III represents exhalation of pure alveolar gas. This usually has a minimal upward slope; one reason for this is that alveoli with longer time constants empty later and have a higher concentration of CO_2. Phase IV represents inspiration.

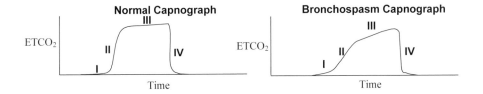

1. Thompson JE, Jaffe MB. Capnographic waveforms in the mechanically ventilated patient. *Respiratory Care* 2005; 50(1): 100-9.
2. Bhavani-Shankar K, *et al.* Capnometry and anaesthesia. *Can J Anaesth* 1992; 39(6): 617-32.

A22 B

In a randomised controlled trial comparing sedation holds with a standard infusion regime, reduced durations of mechanical ventilation (4.9 vs. 7.3 days) and ICU stay (6.4 vs. 9.9 days) were observed in the sedation hold group. Since this group was 'awake' for a greater proportion of the time, neurological assessment was facilitated, and fewer CT brain scans were required to rule out intracerebral causes for reduced consciousness. No reduction in mortality was demonstrated. Since propofol has a shorter context-sensitive half-life than midazolam, its effects wore off more quickly during the sedation hold, and the infusion was restarted sooner when compared with the midazolam group. Hence, the drug-sparing effect was greater with midazolam.

1. Kress JP, *et al.* Daily interruption of sedative infusions in critically ill patients undergoing mechanical ventilation. *N Engl J Med* 2000; 342: 1471-7.

A23 E

There is a lack of high quality evidence to guide the use of vena cava filters. Although filters used in conjunction with anticoagulation have been shown to reduce the incidence of pulmonary embolism (PE) compared with anticoagulation alone, they increase the incidence of deep vein thrombosis (DVT) and confer no long-term mortality benefit. In patients with DVT, vena cava filters alone are inferior to anticoagulation for the prevention of PE. The risk of recurrence or extension of venous thromboembolism (VTE) is especially high (40%) in the first month following diagnosis of a clot, and a filter should be considered in such patients if they require major surgery precluding anticoagulation during this period. The same applies to heavily pregnant patients who develop VTE shortly before delivery. Hypercoagulable patients (e.g. underlying malignancy, antiphospholipid syndrome) should first be treated with adequate and then supranormal levels of anticoagulation before being considered for a vena cava filter; such patients are especially prone to recurrent DVT if a filter is placed.

1. British Committee for Standards in Haematology: Writing group: Baglin TP, Brush J, Streiff M. Guidelines on use of vena cava filters. *British Journal of Haematology* 2006; 134: 590-5.

A24 E

A variety of drugs can precipitate the syndrome including monoamine oxidase inhibitors, tricyclics, lithium, valproate, fentanyl, ondansetron and sympathomimetic drugs of abuse. Symptoms and signs may include: altered mental status (hallucinations, restlessness, confusion, coma); neuromuscular signs (clonus, myoclonus, ataxia, hyper-reflexia); autonomic instability (hyperthermia, tachycardia, swings in blood pressure). Cyproheptadine is a serotonin antagonist which has been used in the treatment of the serotonin syndrome. This is a dose-related phenomenon, unlike the neuroleptic malignant syndrome. The latter is an idiosyncratic drug reaction to dopamine antagonists characterised by extrapyramidal signs (lead pipe rigidity, bradykinesia), autonomic instability and fluctuating consciousness. Unlike the serotonin syndrome, onset of the neuroleptic malignant syndrome is usually gradual over a period of several days.

1. Boyer EW, Shannon M. The serotonin syndrome. *New Engl J Med* 2005; 352: 1112-20.

A25 E

Ranson's criteria for acute pancreatitis predict mortality. They are validated for alcoholic pancreatitis and are often used as a guide to severity (Table 1).

Table 1. Ranson's criteria.

On presentation	Developing in the first 24h
Age >55 years	Haematocrit fall >10%
Aspartate aminotransferase >250U/L	Arterial PO_2 <8kPa (<60mmHg)
Blood glucose >11.2mmol/L	Base deficit >-4mmol/L
White cell count >16x10^3/mm^3	Estimated fluid sequestration >6L
Serum lactate dehydrogenase >350U/l	Urea rise >5mg/L

Mortality: 0-2 criteria 2%, 3-4 15%, 5-6 40%, 7-8 100%

1. Ranson, JH, Rifkind, KM, Roses, DF, *et al.* Prognostic signs and the role of operative management in acute pancreatitis. *Surg Gynecol Obstet* 1974; 139: 69.

A26   C

Wolff-Parkinson-White syndrome (WPW) is characterised by an accessory conduction pathway between the atria and ventricles, capable of faster speeds of conduction. The resting ECG is characterised by a short PR interval and a delta wave (a slurred upstroke of the QRS complex caused by ventricular pre-excitation). The commonest accessory pathway is the bundle of Kent. The PR interval in WPW is short because the accessory pathway conducts the atrial impulse faster than the atrioventricular node. The QRS complex is broad with a slurred upstroke because initial ventricular depolarisation via the accessory pathway does not travel in the specialised ventricular conducting system and is therefore slower.

1. Holt A. Management of cardiac arrhythmias. In: *Oh's Intensive Care Manual*, 5th Ed. Bersten AD, Soni N, Eds. Edinburgh: Butterworth-Heinemann, 2003: 173-74.

A27   A

Various drug combinations may be required to maintain homeostasis prior to organ harvesting depending on the condition of the patient and the requirements of the transplant team. Discussion of the deceased's wishes with relatives is mandatory, however, since a clearly stated prior objection from the patient would preclude any organ harvesting.

1. Streat S. Organ donation. In: *Oh's Intensive Care Manual*, 5th Ed. Bersten AD, Soni N, Eds. Edinburgh: Butterworth-Heinemann, 2003: 965-71.

A28   E

Case series of ventilated patients with idiopathic pulmonary fibrosis show a gloomy outlook. Non-invasive ventilation is ineffective in preventing the need for intubation and mechanical ventilation (in contrast to patients with obstructive lung disease). The commonest cause for deterioration in respiratory function is progression of the disease process (47%), followed by pneumonia (31%). In one case series, survival of ventilated patients to ICU discharge was 27% (4/15), but only two patients survived to hospital discharge [1]. In another series (including patients who did not require mechanical ventilation), 61% survived to hospital discharge, but 90% of these were dead within 6 months [2]. Presence of an infectious cause of deterioration does not seem to improve the outlook even if treated with appropriate antibiotics. FEV_1 was similar between survivors and non-survivors.

1.   Blivet S, *et al.* Outcome of patients with idiopathic pulmonary fibrosis admitted to the ICU for respiratory failure. *Chest* 2001; 120(1): 209-12.
2.   Saydain G, *et al.* Outcome of patients with idiopathic pulmonary fibrosis admitted to the Intensive Care Unit. *Am J Respir Crit Care Med* 2002; 166: 839-42.

A29   B

This patient has acute severe asthma with life-threatening features. Nebulised ipratropium bromide produces additional bronchodilation when given with a ß2 agonist and should be given 4-6 hourly. Intravenous magnesium sulphate 2g should be given if the patient fails to respond to initial treatment as in this case. Intravenous aminophylline has not been shown to be of general benefit in a meta-analysis of trial data, but may be of use in selected cases of life-threatening asthma unresponsive to initial treatments. Oral prednisolone is as effective as intravenous hydrocortisone assuming the patient is able to swallow. Heliox has not been shown to improve outcome in acute severe asthma, although when used as the driving gas for nebulised therapy it may improve drug delivery to the small airways. A systematic review of the available evidence concluded that Heliox did not alter outcome and could not be recommended in the emergency treatment of acute severe asthma [1]. It is not recommended in the latest British Thoracic Society guidelines [2].

1. Rodrigo GJ, *et al.* Use of helium-oxygen mixtures in the treatment of acute severe asthma: a systematic review. *Chest* 2003; 123: 891-6.
2. British Thoracic Society, Scottish Intercollegiate Guidelines Network. British guideline on the management of asthma. Available online at: http://www.brit-thoracic.org.uk.

A30   D

Three randomised controlled trials have investigated proning in ARDS. Gattinoni *et al* [1] could not demonstrate improvement in patients randomised to proning for an average of 7 h/d for 10 days. Post hoc analysis suggested that mortality at 10 days was lower in the quartile of patients with the lowest PaO_2/FiO_2 ratios, and in those with the highest Simplified Acute Physiology Scores (SAPS) II; these benefits did not persist following ICU discharge however. Guerin *et al* [2] similarly could not demonstrate a 28-day mortality benefit in patients with acute respiratory failure (the majority with ARDS/acute lung injury [ALI]) randomised to prone ventilation instituted shortly after intubation and applied for a mean of 8.6h/day for a mean of 4.1 days. Most recently, Mancebo *et al* [3] randomised ARDS/ALI patients to proning for 20h/day starting within 48 hours of tracheal intubation and continuing until preset weaning criteria were met. Although a 15% absolute reduction in ICU mortality was suggested, this did not reach statistical significance. Although these trials have not proven proning to be beneficial, they were not adequately powered to confirm a lack of benefit. Therefore, it cannot be categorically stated that proning does not improve outcome: "absence of evidence is not evidence of absence".

1. Gattinoni L, *et al.* Effect of prone positioning on the survival of patients with acute respiratory failure. *N Engl J Med* 2001; 345: 568-73.
2. Guerin C, *et al.* Effects of systematic prone positioning in hypoxemic acute respiratory failure: a randomized controlled trial. *JAMA* 2004; 292: 2379-87.
3. Mancebo J, *et al.* A multicenter trial of prolonged prone ventilation in severe acute respiratory distress syndrome. *Am J Respir Crit Care Med* 2006; 173: 1233-9.

A31   D

This lady has poor oxygen saturation, bibasal crackles on chest auscultation and systemic hypotension as well as a very fast (>150bpm) ventricular rate. She is therefore considered to be high risk. Although there is a risk of embolisation when cardioverting a patient with longstanding atrial fibrillation (AF) who is not anticoagulated (6.8%), this is outweighed by the need for urgent heart rate control. Rate control with metoprolol or digoxin would be a reasonable alternative to cardioversion in a less unwell patient, since long-term maintenance of sinus rhythm is unlikely in a patient of this age with longstanding AF, and rate control has been shown to be at least as effective as rhythm control with regard to long-term mortality. There is no difference in the incidence of embolic problems between chemical or electrical cardioversion; the latter is faster and should be employed in this case.

1. Advanced Life Support Provider Manual, 4th Ed. Resuscitation Council UK, 2004.
2. Bjerkelund CJ, Orning OM. The efficacy of anticoagulation therapy in preventing embolism related to DC electrical conversion of atrial fibrillation. *Am J Cardiol* 1969; 23: 208-16.

A32   A

The intra-aortic balloon pump is typically inserted in a retrograde fashion via the femoral artery, and advanced up the descending aorta until the balloon is just distal to the left subclavian artery. It may be inserted via the subclavian artery and advanced in an anterograde direction, however. The distal end of the balloon must lie above the renal arteries to avoid compromising renal artery perfusion. The balloon inflates during diastole, beginning with the closure of the aortic valve (marked by the dicrotic notch on the arterial pressure waveform). It deflates during isovolumetric contraction sufficiently before ejection to allow diastolic pressure to fall to a lower level than would occur without the IABP pumping. Systolic and diastolic blood pressures usually decrease slightly with IABP use, but the augmented diastolic pressure (the peak pressure produced during IABP inflation in diastole) is higher, increasing coronary perfusion. Deflation of the balloon reduces afterload and reduces cardiac work and oxygen demand.

1.   Boehmer JP, Popjes E. Cardiac failure: mechanical support strategies. *Crit Care Med* 2006; 34(9): S268-78.

A33   B

Full blood count may reveal thrombocytopenia; this may have contributed to a haemorrhagic stroke, and might be a contraindication to thrombolysis. Cardiac arrhythmias are commonly associated with stroke, especially atrial fibrillation. In addition, cardiac ischaemia and myocardial infarction are commonly precipitated as a result of excessive catecholamine release. Hypoglycaemia is a common mimic of stroke, and resolution of symptoms may be swift and complete with treatment of neuroglycopaenia. Hyperglycaemia increases secondary brain injury and should be normalised in the acute setting. Early CT brain scan is mandatory to exclude haemorrhage, allowing antiplatelet treatment and possibly thrombolysis to be administered. Chest X-ray is rarely helpful in the acute phase of stroke unless the patient has respiratory symptoms.

1.   Khaja AM, Grotta JC. Established treatments for acute ischaemic stroke. *Lancet* 2007; 369: 319-30.

A34   A

Myasthenia gravis commonly presents in women in their fourth or fifth decades. Ocular symptoms are the commonest initial presentation. An association with other autoimmune diseases (including hyperthyroidism) is common. Autonomic disturbances are not a feature (although muscarinic symptoms may develop with over-treatment with acetylcholinesterase inhibitors). Botulism may present with cranial nerve signs including diplopia and ptosis. A flaccid descending paralysis is also classical. It is caused by presynaptic inhibition of acetylcholine release by neurotoxins A, B and E which may be ingested or contaminate wounds. Unlike myasthenia gravis, antimuscarinic features are also typical, including dry mouth, mydriasis, constipation and urinary retention. Lyme disease is a tick-borne infection with the spirochete, *Borrelia burgdorferi*. It is characterised by low-grade fever, erythema migrans and myalgia/arthralgia; it is rare in the UK. Charcot-Marie-Tooth disease is an inherited cause of peripheral neuropathy which manifests early in life with distal leg weakness. Guillain-Barré syndrome may present with cranial nerve involvement (particularly the Miller-Fisher variant), but usually begins with distal onset weakness, sensory symptoms and autonomic involvement. An antecedent history of viral or bacterial infection is also common.

1. Drachman DB. Myasthenia gravis. *New Engl J Med* 1994; 330: 1797-1810.

A35 A

Several studies including a single centre randomised controlled trial [1] have compared the relative merits of intermittent haemodialysis (IHD) and continuous renal replacement therapy (CRRT) in the intensive care setting. IHD is much more efficient at removing urea (clearance 198ml/min) than continuous veno-venous haemodiafiltration (30ml/min) and, therefore, requires a much shorter time frame, and is less labour-intensive for the ICU staff. Volumes of fluid in excess of 500ml/h can safely be removed with IHD. Despite concerns regarding haemodynamic instability, IHD was not associated with any greater instability or use of vasopressors/inotropes than CRRT in this study. No mortality benefit has been shown in any methodologically sound prospective study to support one form of renal replacement therapy over another. This has been confirmed in a recent large meta-analysis [2].

1. Uehlinger DE, *et al.* Comparison of continuous and intermittent renal replacement therapy for acute renal failure. *Nephrol Dial Transplant* 2005; 20: 1630-7.
2. Pannu N, *et al.* Renal replacement therapy in patients with acute renal failure: a systematic review. *JAMA* 2008; 299(7): 793-805.

A36 C

Striated muscle breakdown releases large quantities of uric acid, potassium, creatine kinase and phosphate. Creatinine is also a component of muscle and is elevated. Phosphate binds with calcium in the extracellular fluid and the combined product may precipitate in the tissues;

mild hypocalcaemia is often seen early in the course of rhabdomyolysis as a consequence. Later on, in the recovery phase, this calcium is mobilised from the tissues and returned to the extracellular space; hence, calcium supplementation should be avoided unless ionised levels are dangerously low.

1. Baker SW, McCutchan HJ. Rhabdomyolysis: case report and discussion. *The Internet Journal of Emergency and Intensive Care Medicine* 2003; 7(1).

A37   A

N-acetylcysteine (NAC) provides complete protection against hepatotoxicity if given within 12 hours of a non-staggered overdose. Patients at higher risk include those with a history of chronic alcohol consumption and those taking enzyme-inducing drugs such as phenytoin and carbamazepine. NAC may be continued indefinitely at 150mg/kg/day in cases of acute liver failure until improvement occurs or a transplant is obtained, although there is limited evidence for the efficacy of this approach. A pH of <7.3 after adequate fluid resuscitation is a King's College Hospital criterion for referral for liver transplantation. A raised prothrombin time is the most sensitive prognostic marker; 50% of patients with a prothrombin time of >36s at 36 hours will develop acute liver failure.

1. Dargan PI, Jones AL. Acetaminophen poisoning: an update for the intensivist. *Crit Care* 2002, 6: 108-10.

A38   C

Disseminated intravascular coagulation (DIC) may result from a number of disparate disease states including sepsis, trauma, obstetric complications, envenomation and burns. The hallmarks of the condition are depletion of clotting factors, thrombocytopaenia and increased circulating fibrin degradation products. The initial insult may be release of tissue thromboplastin activating the extrinsic pathway (e.g. burns, crush injury, retained dead foetus). Alternatively, endothelial damage may activate the intrinsic pathway (e.g. sepsis, vasculitis, burns). A chronic, compensated form of DIC may exist in malignancy (especially promyelocytic leukaemia and prostatic adenocarcinoma) where increased coagulation is compensated for by increased clotting factor production. In such cases, tests of coagulation and fibrinogen levels may be near-normal, although fibrin degradation products will still be elevated. Schistocytes (fragmented red cells) are found in DIC, especially chronic forms. Target cells are red cells with a 'bullseye' microscopic appearance and are found in hyposplenism, certain haemoglobinopathies and liver disease.

1. Vasani K. Disseminated intravascular coagulation: a review with experience from an intensive care unit in India. *J Postgrad Med* 1992; 38(4): 186-93.

A39 C

Endoscopic therapy is the treatment of choice providing a suitably experienced operator is available. This allows precise diagnosis as well as treatment. Somatostatin is appropriate pharmacological therapy if endoscopy is not an option and known varices are present. Propranolol is indicated for prophylaxis but not treatment of an acute variceal bleed. Balloon tamponade is highly effective at controlling bleeding (90% of cases), but is associated with a high rate of further bleeding (50%), and complications such as oesophageal ulceration and aspiration pneumonia. Both endoscopic banding and sclerotherapy are effective in stopping variceal bleeding. Banding has been shown to be superior to sclerotherapy in eradicating bleeding [1], and may be associated with increased survival. Sclerotherapy is also associated with an increased risk of bacteraemia.

1. Laine L, Cook D. Endoscopic ligation compared with sclerotherapy for treatment of esophageal variceal bleeding. A meta-analysis. *Ann Intern Med* 1995; 123(4): 280-7.
2. Qureshi W, *et al.* ASGE guideline: the role of endoscopy in the management of variceal hemorrhage, updated July 2005. *Gastrointest Endosc* 2005; 62(5): 651-5.

A40   A

The silhouette sign is the absence of the normally well-defined interface between lung and soft tissue structures. If the air in the lung at the interface is removed (e.g. consolidation), the radiographic boundary will disappear. Pleural capping is the obliteration of the medial aspect of the left upper lobe seen in some cases of aortic dissection. Bat's wing shadowing is perihilar oedema of the lung fields adjacent to the heart seen in congestive cardiac failure. Air bronchograms are (radiolucent) intrapulmonary airways made visible by their passage through a zone of (radio-opaque) consolidation. Wedge-shaped shadows may represent an area of infarcted lung in pulmonary embolism.

1.   Hodgkinson DW, O'Driscoll BR. Chest. In: *ABC of Emergency Radiology*. Nicholson DA, Driscoll PA, Eds. Cambridge: BMJ Publishing Group, 1995: 47-56.

A41   A

Cocaine causes a hypercoagulable state by decreasing protein C and antithrombin III levels, and increases platelet activation. These changes predispose to arterial thrombosis which may cause stroke, myocardial infarction or even aortic thrombosis. Cocaine can cause ischaemic stroke secondary either to cerebral vasospasm or thrombosis. Haemorrhagic stroke may also occur as part of a hypertensive crisis, especially in the presence of Berry aneurysms or arteriovenous malformations. Accumulation of dopamine in the basal ganglia as a consequence of repeated cocaine ingestion may lead to a variety of movement disorders including choreoathetosis, dystonias and akathisia. Cocaine has immunogenic properties, and may act as a hapten which triggers a hypersensitivity pneumonitis when combined with albumin or globulins. This is known as 'crack lung' and is characterised by fever, dyspnoea, wheezing and diffuse interstitial infiltrates. Pulmonary infarction, haemorrhage and asthma are other pulmonary manifestations of cocaine abuse, which affect 25% of users. Bowel ischaemia is the commonest gastrointestinal complication of cocaine use secondary to vasospasm of the mesenteric circulation. Gastroduodenal perforation is a well recognised consequence; gastric stasis also contributes by prolonging exposure to gastric acid.

1. Chanti CM, Lucas CE. Cocaine and the critical care challenge. *Crit Care Med* 2003; 31(6): 1851-9.

A42 C

Phencyclidine (PCP) acts on various neurotransmitter systems and has a variable clinical presentation. Hypertension is common, and agitation with pinpoint pupils should raise suspicion of the diagnosis. Psychiatric phenomena are common including hallucinations, delusions and agitation; trauma is common as a consequence. Based on the data given, urinary acidification will increase the ionised proportion of the drug and thus enhance renal elimination. Although this has been advocated as a treatment, 90% of the drug is metabolised by the liver, therefore the effect of even enhanced urinary elimination is minor. Lipid-soluble drugs can cross the blood-brain barrier and the placenta. Haemodialysis is likely to be ineffective for a drug with a large volume of distribution that is significantly protein-bound and has minimal renal elimination. Hypertension is likely given the sympathomimetic and serotonergic properties of the drug, and is a common feature of PCP ingestion. Benzodiazepines and/or combined alpha- and beta-blockade may be required. It can be assumed that a highly lipid-soluble drug will have a large volume of distribution that will considerably exceed total body water.

1. Bey T, Patel A. Phencyclidine intoxication and adverse effects: a clinical and pharmacological review of an illicit drug. *California J Emerg Med* 2007; 8(1): 9-14.

A43 D

Systemic vascular resistance falls by 30% in early pregnancy. This is opposed by an increase in the activity of the renin-angiotensin-aldosterone system which retains volume and sodium. Cardiac output also increases; the net effect is a modest decrease in blood pressure, with systolic falling to a lesser extent than diastolic. The major benefit of treating hypertension in pregnancy is to prevent end-organ damage in the mother. There is little benefit to the foetus except when treating extremely high blood pressure. Pregnancy-induced hypertension usually supervenes in the latter stages of pregnancy, and hypertension detected before 20 weeks is likely to be chronic essential hypertension rather than pregnancy-induced.

1. Vidaeff AC, Carroll MA, Ramin SM. Acute hypertensive emergencies in pregnancy. *Crit Care Med* 2005; 33(10): S307-12.

A44 C

Intubation of the pre-eclamptic patient is fraught with danger. The potentially difficult airway of pregnancy is accentuated, with facial and tongue oedema making direct laryngoscopy difficult. The pressor response to intubation may cause a further rise in blood pressure risking stroke (or worsening of intracerebral haemorrhage in this case). This response can be attenuated with short-acting opiates such as alfentanil. Although intravenous lignocaine may be effective in this regard, it can cross the placenta and may accumulate in the acidic foetal environment ('ion trapping' due to ionisation of the basic drug). Sodium nitroprusside is very effective in lowering blood pressure, but may cause a precipitous drop worsening cerebral perfusion. It has several undesirable side effects including lactic acidosis and cyanide toxicity. Its use is therefore reserved for hypertension that does not settle with other agents (e.g. labetalol). The foetus is not compromised and while early delivery may be advised, a history suggestive of extradural haematoma is given; in this case early CT brain scan and evacuation of haematoma could be life-saving. Involvement of senior obstetric, intensive care and neurosurgical specialists would be mandatory in this case.

1. Munnur U, de Boisblanc B, Suresh MS. Airway problems in pregnancy. *Crit Care Med* 2005; 33(10): S259-68.
2. Torr GJ, James MFM. The role of the anaesthetist in the management of pre-eclampsia. *Update in Anaesthesia* 1998; Issue 9: Article 4.

A45 E

Dobutamine is primarily a β-1 agonist which increases cardiac contractility and heart rate. It also has significant β-2 agonist activity which causes peripheral vasodilatation and a fall in systemic vascular resistance. It has a half-life of 2 minutes and is metabolised by catechol-O-methyl transferase (COMT) to inactive metabolites. Both systolic and diastolic function are improved in heart failure, leading to an increase in cardiac index and a fall in left ventricular end-diastolic pressure (LVEDP). It increases myocardial oxygen demand, but is often indicated in heart failure secondary to ischaemic heart disease (IHD), and is used as a form of myocardial stress testing for risk stratification of patients with symptoms of IHD.

1. Sasada M, Smith S. *Drugs in Anaesthesia & Intensive Care*, 3rd Ed. New York: Oxford University Press, 2003.
2. Tennyson H, *et al.* Treatment of post-resuscitation myocardial dysfunction: aortic counterpulsation versus dobutamine. *Resuscitation* 2002; 54: 69-75.

A46 E

The liver and splanchnic circulation normally account for 25-30% of cardiac output, but this falls dramatically in critical illness due to splanchnic vasoconstriction. Flow-limited drugs with a high extraction ratio such as midazolam will accumulate significantly. Remifentanil is metabolised by non-specific plasma esterases and can be used as normal. Drugs with a low extraction ratio are metabolism-limited (they depend on saturable enzyme systems for metabolism) rather than flow-limited, and will not be affected by reduced liver blood flow, unless the reduction is so severe as to cause hepatocellular injury and reduced enzyme function.

1. Short TG, Hood GC. Pharmacokinetics, pharmacodynamics and drug monitoring in critical illness. In: *Oh's Intensive Care Manual*, 5th Ed. Bersten AD, Soni N, Eds. Edinburgh: Butterworth-Heinemann, 2003: 814-6.
2. Shelly MP, *et al.* Failure of critically ill patients to metabolise midazolam. *Anaesthesia* 1987; 42(6): 619-26.

A47   D

During spontaneous breathing the maximum inspiratory flow rate can exceed 30L/min for brief periods. A standard Hudson-type mask will therefore not supply a constant fraction of inspired oxygen (FiO_2) unless the flow rate of oxygen through the connecting tubing exceeds 30L/min, since air will be entrained at a variable ratio throughout the respiratory cycle. The Venturi effect (based on the Bernoulli principle) states that when a gas passes through a constriction the pressure falls, thus allowing a second gas to be entrained. The Venturi mask has a constriction through which oxygen flows, entraining a fixed ratio of air dependent on the size of the constriction and the flow of oxygen. This allows a high volume of gas of a known FiO_2 to be available for inspiration (fixed performance). Mouth breathing with nasal cannulae allows a Venturi effect to occur in the nasopharynx with oxygen-enriched air being entrained from the nose during inspiration (although performance is variable). Masks such as the Venturi and Hudson are loose fitting and have holes permitting ready elimination of waste gases; they do not significantly increase dead space. Anaesthetic face masks have a tight seal with the patient's face and may be bulky, increasing dead space, although this is not usually clinically significant in adult practice.

1.   Masks. In: *Essentials of Anaesthetic Equipment*, 2nd Ed. Al-Shaikh B, Stacey S. London: Churchill-Livingstone, 2002: 73-9.

A48   B

As a rule, oral metronidazole is first-line therapy for uncomplicated *C. difficile* infection since it is generally effective and cheap. However, it is associated with a significant relapse rate of up to 25% in the first 10 days following cessation of therapy. Patients deemed at increased risk of an adverse outcome include those with a high white cell count ($>20 \times 10^9$/L) and creatinine $>200\mu$mol/L (2.26mg/dL). In addition, patients over the age of 65 are at greater risk of serious complications such as toxic megacolon, perforation and death in the event of a recurrence. Oral vancomycin is the treatment of choice for patients with these risk factors since resistance is rare and it reaches high concentrations in the colon. In contrast, intravenous vancomycin is ineffective since it has poor penetration of the colon. Intravenous metronidazole is effective, however, and may be useful if an ileus preventing the enteral administration of drugs is present. Nasojejunal faecal replacement has been used with some success in treating chronic *C. difficile* infection, where it re-colonises the patient's colon with normal flora. It has no place in the management of acute infection however.

1.   Kuijper EJ, van Dissel JT, Wilcox MH. *Clostridium difficile*: changing epidemiology and new treatment options. *Current Opinion in Infectious Diseases* 2007; 20: 376-83.

A49   B

A large multi-centre snapshot study collected data on all adverse incidents reported in 205 ICUs worldwide over a 24-hour period [1]. The overall incident rate was 38.8 events per 100 patient days. The commonest adverse incident was related to lines, drains and catheters (14.5/100 patient days). Medication errors were the next most frequent (10.5/100 patient days), with administration errors (wrong route, dose or drug) almost as common as prescribing errors. Equipment failure accounted for 9.2 events per 1000 patient days, mainly related to infusion pumps. Ventilator dysfunction occurred in 1.9% of all patients receiving mechanical ventilation over the study period. Airway problems including accidental extubation, occlusion and cuff leakage occurred in 3.3/100 patient days, while inappropriate turn-off of alarms had an incidence of 1.3/100 patient days.

1.   Valentin A, *et al.* Patient safety in intensive care: results from the multinational Sentinel Events Evaluation (SEE) study. *Int Care Med* 2006; 32: 1591-8.

A50   D

Tracheomalacia results from ischaemic injury to the trachea followed by chondritis and subsequent destruction and necrosis of supporting tracheal cartilage. This causes the trachea to collapse during expiration but remain patent during inspiration. It may result from tracheostomy or prolonged transtracheal intubation, and may present as failure to wean from mechanical ventilation, or later as exertional dyspnoea. The patient may note that exhalation is difficult while inhalation is easier. Flow-volume loops may show the characteristic pattern of variable intrathoracic obstruction (shown in the question), with a normal inspiratory limb and a flattened expiratory limb. Bronchoscopy and/or dynamic CT scanning demonstrate severe narrowing of the trachea on expiration. For severe cases, management options include tracheal excision, tracheoplasty or stenting. Bronchospasm and interstitial lung diseases typically show characteristic flow-volume loops. Tracheal stenosis presents as a fixed upper airway obstruction with impedence to inspiratory as well as expiratory airflow.

1. Epstein SK. Late complications of tracheostomy. *Respir Care* 2005; 50(4): 542-9.

Paper 1

Type 'K' answers

K51   FTFT

SIADH is characterised by a low plasma sodium, high urinary sodium excretion and a predisposing cause. This commonly includes tumours, central nervous system lesions and pulmonary diseases. SIADH is usually euvolaemic. Although in cases of severe hyponatraemia (sodium <120mmol/l) there may be an excess of total body water of several litres, pitting oedema is not usually a feature. This is more in keeping with causes of secondary hyperaldosteronism such as cardiac, renal and hepatic failure where salt and water are retained.

1.   Bersten AD, Soni N. *Oh's Intensive Care Manual*, 5th Ed. Edinburgh: Butterworth-Heinemann, 2003.

K52   TTFT

Normal serum magnesium levels are 0.6-1mmol/L. Absorption of dietary magnesium occurs in the terminal ileum, and excretion is via the kidney; most is reabsorbed in the proximal tubule and thick ascending limb of the loop of Henle. Hypomagnesaemia occurs through malabsorption, diarrhoea, malnutrition, renal disease and a variety of drugs (diuretics, cisplatin, pentamidine). Diabetics lose magnesium through osmotic diuresis, alcoholics through a combination of osmotic diuresis and malnutrition. The prevalence of hypomagnesaemia is 2% in the general population but 50-60% in ICU patients. Symptoms and signs are legion and non-specific; flushing is a sign of hypermagnesaemia.

1. Dube L, Granry J-C. The therapeutic use of magnesium in anesthesiology, intensive care and emergency medicine: a review. *Can J Anaesth* 2003; 50: 732-46.

K53 TFTT

Microshock is caused when a small current passes directly to the myocardium, for example via a faulty intracardiac catheter. Although the current may be small, the current density may be high at the site of injury, precipitating ventricular fibrillation. Risk of ventricular fibrillation increases with current density in the myocardium, and is greatest at lower current frequencies (maximal around 50Hz). An oesophageal probe could theoretically conduct sufficient current to the left atrium to cause microshock. Type CF equipment has electrodes which may contact the heart directly and has a maximum leakage current of <50µA even if operating with a single fault.

1. Davis PD, Parbrook GD, Kenny GN. *Basic Physics and Measurement in Anaesthesia*, 4th Ed. Oxford: Butterworth Heinemann, 2002.

K54 TTTF

Two randomised controlled trials have shown a significantly higher incidence of good neurological outcome in patients treated with therapeutic hypothermia compared with normothermic controls both at the time of hospital discharge (49% vs 26%) [1] and 6 months later (55% vs 39%) [2]. It is generally accepted that fast and immediate cooling to the target temperature confers the greatest benefit. Both trials used 12-24 hours as the period of hypothermia; the exact optimum time is still a matter for debate.

1. Bernard SA, *et al.* Treatment of comatose survivors of out-of-hospital cardiac arrest with induced hypothermia. *New Engl J Med* 2002; 346: 557-63.
2. The Hypothermia After Cardiac Arrest Study Group: mild therapeutic hypothermia to improve neurological outcome after cardiac arrest. *New Engl J Med* 2002; 346: 549-56.

K55 FTTF

The history is suggestive of pulmonary contusion. This develops following trauma as a combination of shear stress, bursting forces and pulmonary vascular damage with secondary alveolar haemorrhage. Initial chest X-ray commonly displays clear lung fields, with opacities taking several hours to appear. A CT scan has much greater sensitivity and will show evidence of pulmonary contusion immediately post-injury. Haemorrhage into the affected lung may continue for 24-48 hours, and contusions resolve after about 7 days. There is no place for prophylactic steroids or antibiotics, although ventilator-acquired pneumonia commonly supervenes. Ventilation with the non-injured side dependent may improve oxygenation by increasing blood flow to the good (ventilated) lung, reducing the shunt fraction. Mortality is around 15% overall, but this increases with the size of contusion, patient age, and presence of other injuries.

1. Cohn SM. Pulmonary contusion: review of the clinical entity. *Journal of Trauma-Injury Infection & Critical Care* 1997; 42(5): 973-9.

K56 TFTF

The major mechanisms of injury in blunt abdominal trauma are deceleration and compression, both of which are present in this case. Compression from a seatbelt can cause subcapsular haematoma to solid organs, and can cause increased intraluminal pressure and rupture of hollow viscera. Deceleration causes shearing between free and fixed structures, classically a hepatic tear along the ligamentum teres and intimal injuries to the renal arteries as well as mesenteric tears. A normal amylase at presentation is neither sensitive nor specific in ruling out pancreatic injury. A raised AST or ALT (>130IU/L) should raise suspicion of hepatic injury. Seatbelt marks increase the likelihood of small intestinal rupture. Hypotensive resuscitation is not supported by high quality evidence in blunt abdominal trauma.

1. Salomone JA. Blunt abdominal trauma. Available: http://www.emedicine.com/emerg/topic1.htm. Last accessed 20 November 2008.

K57   TTFF

The GCS after initial resuscitation is the most important prognostic indicator. The motor component is the most useful aspect of this. The Marshall grading system of CT brain appearance in diffuse axonal injury comprises grades I-IV which correlate with mortality (Table 1). The Medical Research Council CRASH trial showed that a 48-hour infusion of IV methylprednisolone in patients with a head injury and GCS of 14 or less was associated with an increase in 14-day mortality compared with placebo (21.1% vs. 17.9%).

Table 1. The Marshall grading system.

Category of diffuse injury	Definition	Mortality (%)
I	No visible intracranial injury	10
II	Cisterns present. Midline shift 0-5mm and small, high, or mixed density lesions <25cc	14
III	Cisterns compressed or absent + I or II	34
IV	Midline shift >5mm + I, II or III	56

1.   Helmy A, Vizcaychipi M, Gupta AK. Traumatic brain injury: intensive care management. *Br J Anaesth* 2007; 99 (1): 32-42.

2.   Marshall LF, Marshall SB, Klauber MR, *et al.* The diagnosis of head injury requires a classification based on computed axial tomography. *J Neurotrauma* 1992; 9(Suppl 1): S287-92.

K58   FTTF

Typical CSF findings in Guillain-Barré syndrome are an elevated protein concentration (normal range is 0.2-0.4g/L), normal glucose and no elevation of white cell count (an elevated white cell count should cast doubt on the diagnosis). Oligoclonal bands are characteristic of (but not specific to) demyelinating disease.

1. Winer JB. Clinical review: Guillain-Barré syndrome. *BMJ* 2008; 337: a671.

K59   FTFF

The history of seizure, headache and neurological deficit post-endarterectomy suggests cerebral hyperperfusion syndrome. This is seen when blood flow is restored to part of the brain where previously it was poor, and normal autoregulatory mechanisms are ineffective. The peak incidence is around day 5 post-operation. It is more common in hypertensive patients, and requires pharmacological treatment (unlike ischaemic stroke where blood pressure is generally left untreated in the acute phase). If left untreated, cerebral oedema and haemorrhagic stroke may occur. A CT brain scan is required to exclude stroke. If treating blood pressure, agents such as labetalol or clonidine are preferred to nitrates which cause cerebral vasodilatation.

1. Adhiyaman V, Alexander S. Cerebral hyperperfusion syndrome following carotid endarterectomy. *Q J Med* 2007; 100(4): 239-44.

K60   FFTF

The brachial artery runs medial to the biceps brachii tendon but lateral to the median nerve. The femoral sheath contains (from medial to lateral) the femoral canal, vein and artery. The femoral nerve runs lateral to but outside the sheath. The long saphenous vein runs 2cm anterior and superior to the medial malleolus.

1. Erdmann AG. *Concise Anatomy for Anaesthesia.* London; San Francisco: Greenwich Medical Media, 2004.

K61   FTFF

Tight glycaemic control has been shown to improve the survival and neurological outcome of patients with traumatic brain injury (TBI) [1]. The incidence of deep vein thrombosis in isolated TBI is around 3%. The timing of initiation of anticoagulant thromboprophylaxis is controversial, but generally would be considered after 72h. Therapeutic hypothermia in TBI has been the subject of several randomised controlled trials and meta-analyses, which have not demonstrated a statistically significant reduction in mortality, although mild hypothermia was found to improve neurological outcome in a recent meta-analysis [2].

1.   Clayton TJ, Nelson RJ, Manara AR. Reduction in mortality from severe head injury following introduction of a protocol for intensive care management. *Br J Anaesth* 2004; 93: 761-7.
2.   Brain Trauma Foundation; American Association of Neurological Surgeons; Congress of Neurological Surgeons; Joint Section on Neurotrauma and Critical Care, AANS/CNS. Guidelines for the management of severe traumatic brain injury. III. Prophylactic hypothermia. *J Neurotrauma* 2007; 24 Suppl 1: S21-5.

K62   TTFF

rFVIIa is licensed for use in the treatment of haemophilia A and B in patients with inhibitory antibodies to factor VIII or IX. It is not licensed for use in trauma. A recent randomised controlled trial compared the use of rFVIIa with placebo in trauma patients who had required a six-unit blood transfusion. In patients with blunt trauma, the treatment arm had a small but significant reduction in the amount of units of blood transfusion required (2.6 units less than the placebo group), and a lesser incidence of massive transfusion (defined as >20 units blood, 14% vs. 33% of patients). This benefit was not shown in patients with penetrating trauma. No mortality benefit has been demonstrated, although numerous anecdotal case reports exist. Pharmacological doses of rVIIa activate Factor X on the surface of platelets leading to the thrombin burst required for clot formation; hence, it will be ineffective in the presence of profound thrombocytopenia. Adequate fibrinogen is also required to ensure formation of a stable clot.

1. Boffard KD, *et al.* Recombinant factor VIIa as adjunctive therapy for bleeding control in severely injured trauma patients: two parallel randomized placebo-controlled double-blind clinical trials. *J Trauma* 2005; 59: 8-15.

K63   TTTT

Type A lactic acidosis refers to hypoperfusion states with excessive anaerobic metabolism and lactate production, while Type B (which has various subtypes) refers to inability of the organs to metabolise a lactate load. Lactate has repeatedly been shown to be of prognostic significance in trauma patients. In one study, all patients with a normalised (<2mmol/L[18mg/dL]) lactate after 24h survived, but only 77.8% survived if normalised by 48h, and 13.6% if still raised at 48h. There is virtually no difference between venous and arterial blood lactate concentrations.

1. Abramson D, *et al.* Lactate clearance and survival following injury. *J Trauma* 1993; 35: 548-89.

K64   TFFF

The history and findings are consistent with a diagnosis of carbon monoxide (COHb) poisoning. This lady had a measured COHb level of 36.4% (data not provided in the question). A standard pulse oximeter measures only two wavelengths of light and falsely interprets COHb as oxyhaemoglobin, overestimating the true arterial oxygen saturation. Many blood gas analysers provide a calculated SaO_2 based on the PaO_2 of oxygen in the blood which is not affected by COHb poisoning; hence, this value is also falsely elevated. True arterial oxygen saturation can be measured using a co-oximeter which uses multiple wavelengths of light. If measured in this case, true SaO_2 would be very low when compared with the falsely elevated SpO_2; this is termed the 'saturation gap'. Since the SaO_2 provided in this question is calculated, however, this is not seen. Indications for hyperbaric oxygen therapy include pregnancy, COHb levels >20%, neurological signs and loss of consciousness. Logistical considerations often preclude its use outside centres with a hyperbaric chamber.

1. Mak TWL, Kam CW, Lai JPS, Tang CMC. Management of carbon monoxide poisoning using oxygen therapy. *Hong Kong Med J* 2000; 6(1): 113-5.

K65   FTFF

Transpulmonary dilution techniques do not require a pulmonary artery catheter, but do require a central line and an arterial cannula. According to the Stewart-Hamilton equation, cardiac output is inversely proportional to the area under the time-temperature curve. A small volume of injectate will tend to overestimate cardiac output since it will thermally equilibrate rapidly with the surrounding environment and generate only a small temperature-time peak. Cold injectate should be ice-cold; the closer the temperature is to blood temperature, the less precise the measurement.

1. Morgan TJ. Haemodynamic monitoring. In: *Oh's Intensive Care Manual*, 5th Ed. Bersten AD, Soni N, Eds. Edinburgh: Butterworth-Heinemann, 2003.

K66   TFTF

Several assumptions are made in determining cardiac output. It is assumed that 70% of the total stroke volume (SV) enters the descending aorta (therefore total SV = measured SV/0.7). The descending aorta is assumed to run parallel to the oesophagus (a divergence of just 10° can cause an error of ~20-30%). SV is obtained by multiplying the velocity-time integral by aortic cross-sectional area, which is assumed to remain constant throughout systole. It is also assumed for this calculation that all red blood cells are moving at maximum velocity. The haematocrit has no bearing on stroke volume determination.

1. Berton C, Cholley B. Equipment review: new techniques for cardiac output measurement - oesophageal Doppler, Fick principle using carbon dioxide, and pulse contour analysis. *Crit Care* 2002; 6(3): 216-21.

K67   TTFT

The half-life of carbon monoxide is: 4h in room air; 1h in 100% oxygen at 1ATM; 25 minutes in 100% oxygen at 3ATM. A carbon monoxide level of >60% is commonly lethal; carbon monoxide poisoning is the commonest cause of death at the scene of a fire. Since the vast majority of oxygen is transported as oxyhaemoglobin, a 50% carboxyhaemoglobin level will reduce oxygen carriage by about 50%. Normal oxygen carriage is around $20mlO_2/100ml$ blood, assuming a PaO_2 of 10kPa and normal haemoglobin concentration, and will fall to $\sim 10mlO_2/100ml$ in the example given. Untreated pneumothorax is an absolute contraindication to hyperbaric therapy, since a 1L pneumothorax at 3ATM will become a 3L pneumothorax at atmospheric pressure following decompression (in accordance with Boyle's law).

1.   Mak TWL, Kam CW, Lai JPS, Tang CMC. Management of carbon monoxide poisoning using oxygen therapy. *Hong Kong Med J* 2000; 6(1): 113-5.

K68   FFFT

Stroke volume can be derived from the area under the systolic portion of the arterial waveform (up to the dicrotic notch). The rate of rise in pressure per unit time (dP/dt) is an index of contractility. Hypovolaemia is suggested by a low dicrotic notch and a narrow waveform, while a steep slope of diastolic decay suggests vasodilatation.

1.   Yentis SM, Hirsch NP, Smith GB. *Anaesthesia and Intensive Care A-Z*, 3rd Ed. London: Butterworth-Heinemann, 2004.

K69   FTFF

The pulse oximeter measures the absorbance of red and infrared light transmitted through tissues. Oxyhaemoglobin absorbs more infrared light (940nm) and allows more red light (660nm) to pass through (and vice versa for deoxyhaemoglobin). The red and infrared diodes flash on and off at least 30 times per second (30Hz) to build up a picture of the pulsatile component of the signal. This pulsatile component (representing arterial blood) is analysed after subtraction of absorbance by the non-pulsatile component (venous blood and tissue). The isobestic point is the wavelength of light at which absorption is the same for oxy- and deoxyhaemoglobin (805nm) regardless of the oxygen saturation of the blood. It serves as a reference point for some types of pulse oximeter. The Lambert-Beer law states that the intensity of transmitted light declines exponentially with increasing concentration or distance through which the light passes. The Hagen-Poiseuille law describes laminar flow of a Newtonian fluid.

1.   Al-Shaikh B, Stacey S. *Essentials of Anaesthetic Equipment*. London: Churchill-Livingstone, 2002.

K70   TFFF

Elevated pulmonary artery pressure and right ventricular dilatation in this clinical context suggests a large pulmonary embolism. The risk of death for pulmonary embolism without right ventricular compromise is less than 1%. This rises to 24% with right ventricular compromise if systemic hypotension is also present. Thrombolysis has been shown to improve right ventricular function but not to reduce the risk of death, and is generally considered for patients with cardiovascular collapse, and is associated with a 3% risk of clinically significant haemorrhage. A left ventricular heave is a reflection of left ventricular hypertrophy, which will not be present in this case as the left ventricle is acutely underfilled, leading to systemic hypotension.

1.   Kinane TB, *et al.* Case 7 2008: a 17-year-old girl with chest pain and haemoptysis. *New Engl J Med* 2008; 358: 941-52.

K71   TFTF

Oesophageal intubation may initially register CO_2 on the capnograph, which disappears over a few breaths (especially if carbonated beverages have been consumed). Endobronchial intubation would cause a gradual rise in end-tidal carbon dioxide ($ETCO_2$), since alveolar minute volume is much-reduced and, therefore, the partial pressure of CO_2 in the blood (and consequently the alveoli) rises. Massive haemorrhage to the point of PEA cardiac arrest would show this trace: with an extremely low cardiac output and blood pressure the alveoli would cease to be perfused and, therefore, alveolar CO_2 and $ETCO_2$ would swiftly fall. Although hyperventilation would in time cause a fall in $ETCO_2$ in line with increased CO_2 elimination from the blood, this would not happen to the extent shown over the course of ten seconds as shown in the capnograph trace.

1. Bhavani-Shankar K, *et al.* Capnometry and anaesthesia. *Can J Anaesth* 1992; 39(6): 617-32.
2. Bhavani-Shankar K. Encyclopedia of capnograms. Available: http://www.capnography.com. Last accessed 16 October 2008.

K72 TTTF

A normal intracranial pressure waveform is shown. Three peaks should be visible: P1 represents transmitted arterial pulsation (the percussion wave); P2 is related to the brain compliance (the tidal wave) and increases as brain compliance falls; and P3 is caused by the closure of the aortic valve (the dicrotic wave). These are distinct from Lundberg waves, which are longer, time-dependent patterns of pressure waves in patients with raised intracranial pressure.

1. Ross N, Eynon CA. Intracranial pressure monitoring. *Current Anaesthesia & Critical Care* 2005; 16: 255-61.

K73 TFFF

Massive haemoptysis is variously defined as blood loss of 100-1000ml in a 24-hour period from the respiratory tract. The volume of blood lost is usually less important than the degree of respiratory compromise; death results from asphyxiation rather than blood loss *per se*. In 90% of cases, bleeding is from the bronchial circulation, which is at much higher (systemic) pressure than the pulmonary circulation. Chest X-ray identifies the source of bleeding in 64-80% of cases but CT scanning has greater sensitivity. The source of bleeding remains occult despite investigations in 5-10% of cases. Nasal septal perforation may suggest Wegener's granulomatosis, a rare cause of massive haemoptysis. Behcet's syndrome is a multisystem disease characterised by recurrent oral aphthous ulcers, genital ulcers and uveitis. Bronchiectasis, tuberculosis and lung cancer are the commonest causes of massive haemoptysis.

1. Lordan JL, Gascoigne A, Corris PA. The pulmonary physician in critical care. Illustrative case 7: assessment and management of massive haemoptysis. *Thorax* 2003; 58: 814-9.

K74 TTFF

The anion gap (AG) is a measure of the difference between unmeasured cations and unmeasured anions in the plasma. This gap is largely explained by unmeasured anionic proteins and organic acids in the blood which contribute to electroneutrality. It is calculated thus: $([Na^+]+[K^+])$ - $([Cl^-]+[HCO_3^-])$, and normal values range from 8-16mmol/L. In the presence of unmeasured volatile acids (lactic acid, ketoacids, ingested acids, uraemia), bicarbonate is lost in buffering and replaced by these unmeasured anions (rather than chloride), hence the AG is raised. In renal or gastrointestinal cases of bicarbonate loss, an increase in chloride ions balances this loss thus maintaining electroneutrality, and the AG is normal. The AG will also be raised if there are low levels of unmeasured cations (calcium, magnesium), and lowered in the presence of low levels of unmeasured anions (principally albumin) or high levels of unmeasured cations (e.g. myeloma paraprotein). Gastric outflow obstruction typically causes a hypochloraemic metabolic alkalosis due to loss of hydrochloric acid. Excessive administration of normal saline can cause a mild hyperchloraemic acidosis; in this case the chloride is within the normal range and the bicarbonate is very low (i.e. a severe acidosis is present).

1. Ganong WF. *Review of Medical Physiology*, 21st Ed. New York: Lange Medical Books, 2003.

K75 TFFT

A tear in the aortic intima allows blood to pass into the media causing dissection. This can originate in the ascending aorta (Stanford Type A) or descending aorta (Type B). Around two thirds originate in the ascending aorta. Hypertension, connective tissue diseases, vasculitis and trauma are risk factors. Transoesophageal echocardiography has a sensitivity of 98% and specificity of 97%, and is especially good for visualising ascending aortic dissection. Medical management involves blood pressure control with reduction of the shear force on the wall of the aorta (dP/dt) with a combination of vasodilators and rate controlling drugs (beta-blockers, verapamil, diltiazem) and is the treatment of choice for uncomplicated Type B dissection. A variety of surgical approaches are indicated for Type A dissection, which carry an operative mortality rate of 15-35% even in centres of excellence.

1. Nienaber CA, Eagle KA. Aortic dissection: new frontiers in diagnosis and management Part II: therapeutic management and follow-up. *Circulation* 2003; 108: 772-8.

K76   FTFT

The Injury Severity Score (ISS) is an anatomical scoring system which divides injuries into six body regions (head, face, chest, abdomen, extremities [including pelvis], external). Injuries in each region are graded according to the Abbreviated Injury Scale (AIS) from 1 (minor injury) to 6 (unsurvivable). The three highest scoring regions have their scores squared and summated to give a maximum of 75 (unsurvivable). A score of 6 in any one region automatically yields an ISS of 75. The ISS correlates linearly with increasing mortality following trauma, but has several limitations. A patient with several wounds to the same body region can only score once for that region; in such a case the ISS may underestimate the severity of their injuries.

1. Baker SP, *et al.* The Injury Severity Score: a method for describing patients with multiple injuries and evaluating emergency care. *J Trauma* 1974; 14: 187-96.

K77   TFTT

The best predictors of increased in-hospital mortality in a large cohort study included: presence of APACHE II-defined comorbid illness, a requirement for >72h mechanical ventilation and failed extubation.

Interestingly, survival rates were also much better in patients with a previous episode of mechanical ventilation (who have presumably therefore demonstrated a 'survival advantage'). The in-hospital mortality rate in patients ventilated for exacerbation of COPD was 15%; patients with COPD ventilated for other reasons (e.g. surgical, heart failure) had a much higher in-hospital mortality (28%). FEV_1 is an important predictor of long-term survival, but does not predict short-term outcome in COPD patients requiring mechanical ventilation.

1.   Nevins ML, Epstein SK. Predictors of outcome for patients with COPD requiring invasive mechanical ventilation. *Chest* 2001; 119: 1840-9.

K78   TFTF

Bronchial artery embolisation is successful in 75-90% of patients, although a rebleeding rate of 10-30% in the first 30 days is seen. Emergency resection is associated with a hospital mortality rate of 4-18%. Patients must have adequate pulmonary reserve to be considered for this procedure. Bronchoscopic lavage with cold saline, epinephrine 1:10,000 or tranexamic acid may be useful and can buy time until a definitive procedure (surgery, embolisation) can be performed. Rigid bronchoscopy has a place in the management of proximal sources of bleeding, but cannot visualise the periphery of the tracheobronchial tree.

1.   Endo S, *et al.* Management of massive hemoptysis in a thoracic surgical unit. *Eur J Cardiothoracic Surg* 2003; 23: 467-72.
2.   Dupree HJ, *et al.* Fiberoptic bronchoscopy of intubated patients with life-threatening hemoptysis. *World J Surg* 2001; 25: 104-7.

K79   FFTF

Various randomised controlled trials have suggested that high levels of PEEP improve both oxygenation and outcome compared with conventional levels. However, in these trials high PEEP was one of a series of measures in a protective ventilation strategy (including ventilating with low tidal volumes). The Assessment of Low tidal Volume and Elevated End-Expiratory Pressure To Obviate Lung Injury (ALVEOLI [1]) trial randomised patients to a protective ventilation strategy with either low (5-12cmH$_2$O) or high (12-24cmH$_2$0) levels of PEEP. No mortality benefit was demonstrated, although indices of oxygenation were improved in the high PEEP group. The rationale for the use of PEEP is that atelectrauma (repeated opening and closing of alveoli) during the respiratory cycle damages the lungs, and may also cause the release of cytokines which fuel the systemic inflammatory response. Application of PEEP aims to prevent this repeated closure and therefore minimise lung damage.

1. The National Heart Lung and Blood Institute ARDS Clinical Trials Network. Higher versus lower positive end-expiratory pressures in patients with the acute respiratory distress syndrome. *N Engl J Med* 2004; 351: 327-36.

K80 FFFT

At slower heart rates there is more time for ventricular filling, which will increase stroke volume. At high heart rates the reverse is true, but cardiac output is increased by the frequency of ventricular systole. Doppler studies suggest that the optimum ventricular rate is around 90bpm at rest as a compromise between stroke volume and heart rate. The atria normally contribute 15-30% of ventricular filling, although this figure becomes higher with age and with impaired left ventricular function where loss of atrial function may lead to a 50% fall in cardiac output. Ischaemic heart disease is the commonest cause of atrial fibrillation; others include rheumatic heart disease, non-rheumatic valvular heart disease, thyrotoxicosis, hypertension, haemochromatosis and sepsis. Successful cardioversion restores a degree of atrial function, but an element of 'stunning' may be present. Atrial mechanical function usually improves over the first 24 hours.

1. Cavaliere F, *et al.* Atrial fibrillation in intensive care units. *Current Anaesthesia & Critical Care* 2006; 17: 367-74.

K81 FFTF

The only absolute contraindications to the use of an intra-aortic balloon pump (IABP) are aortic dissection and clinically significant aortic regurgitation. Refractory angina is a possible indication for use as a bridge to definitive therapy, since one of the primary benefits of the IABP is an increase in coronary perfusion pressure. Severe peripheral vascular disease involving the abdominal aorta, iliac or femoral arteries is a relative contraindication, since distal ischaemia is a risk. Morbid obesity and abdominal aortic aneurysm are also relative contraindications.

1. Boehmer JP, Popjes E. Cardiac failure: mechanical support strategies. *Crit Care Med* 2006; 34(9): S268-78.

K82   TFFF

This man has clinical evidence of a stroke. The CT brain scan has excluded haemorrhage, but failed to show ischaemic changes (which are not usually visible in the first few hours post-stroke). Aspirin 300mg has been shown to reduce recurrence of stroke, death and disability, and should be given to all stroke patients once haemorrhage has been excluded [1]. The evidence base for clopidogrel has not been established in stroke, and this should not be routinely given. Anticoagulation has no benefit in the acute phase of ischaemic stroke (except in special cases such as venous sinus thrombosis) and should not be given. Hypertension is common in acute stroke, and may be pre-existing, and/or elevated due to stress, pain or as a physiological response to brain hypoxia. It should not be actively lowered unless pressures of 220mmHg (systolic) or 120mmHg (diastolic) are reached. If thrombolysis is considered, lower thresholds for treatment exist (185mmHg systolic, 110mmHg diastolic) [2].

1. Royal College of Physicians. National clinical guidelines for stroke, 2nd Ed. Prepared by the Intercollegiate Stroke Working Party. London: RCP, 2004.
2. Adams HP, *et al.* Guidelines for the early management of patients with ischemic stroke: a scientific statement from the Stroke Council of the American Stroke Association. *Stroke* 2003; 34: 1056-83.

K83   FTTF

Encephalopathy is a non-inflammatory diffuse brain dysfunction, caused by intoxication or metabolic dysfunction. Encephalitis is an infection of brain tissue, which is a medical emergency. It is characterised by an acute deterioration in mental status, the presence of focal neurological signs and seizures, and peripheral manifestations of the infectious agent (most commonly viral, e.g. parotitis, myocarditis, lymphadenopathy). Cerebrospinal fluid is rarely normal in encephalitis. A lymphocytic pleocytosis may indicate tuberculosis, while polymerase chain reaction (PCR) testing is extremely sensitive for the detection of viral agents. *Herpes simplex* is the commonest cause of encephalitis.

1. Polhill S, Soni M. Encephalitis in the ICU setting. *Current Anaesthesia & Critical Care* 2007; 18: 107-16.

K84   FFTT

The kidneys require adequate perfusion which is traditionally maintained with a combination of fluids and vasopressors. While ischaemia due to renal hypoperfusion is a cause of acute renal failure (ARF), the majority of cases of ARF in the ICU setting are secondary to sepsis and the systemic inflammatory response despite the presence of adequate blood flow to the kidneys. Low-dose dopamine has been shown to be devoid of any reno-protective effect in such patients [1]. Mannitol is widely used with the premise of 'flushing out' debris from the renal tubules with the aim of reducing the incidence of acute tubular necrosis. There is no good evidence on which to base this usage. Normal saline infusion has been shown to significantly reduce the incidence of post-contrast nephropathy when compared with oral hydration alone [2]. N-acetylcysteine has also been shown to reduce the incidence of this complication [3] and is an appropriate pre-treatment for ICU patients awaiting contrast-requiring investigations.

1. Bellomo R, Chapman M, Finfer S, *et al.* Low-dose dopamine in patients with early renal dysfunction: a placebo-controlled randomised trial: Australian and New Zealand Intensive Care Society (ANZICS) Clinical Trials Group. *Lancet* 2000; 356: 2139-43.
2. Trivedi HS, Moore H, Nasr S, *et al.* A randomized prospective trial to assess the role of saline hydration on the development of contrast nephrotoxicity. *Nephron Clin Pract* 2003; 93: C29-34.
3. Marenzi G, Assanelli E, Marana I, *et al.* N-acetylcysteine and contrast-induced nephropathy in primary angioplasty. *N Engl J Med* 2006; 354: 2773-82.

K85 TFFT

Fulminant hepatic failure is characterised by the development of hepatic encephalopathy with a marked decline in hepatic synthetic function within 28 days of the onset of symptoms in patients without a history of chronic liver disease. The hallmarks of the condition are coagulopathy and encephalopathy. Encephalopathy is graded from I (euphoria/depression, mild confusion) to IV (coma). The coagulopathy should not be corrected in the absence of bleeding or invasive procedures, since it is a useful marker of synthetic function which helps guide the need for transplantation. Mortality without liver transplantation is around 90% for fulminant hepatic failure overall, although hepatitis A and paracetamol poisoning are associated with better survival rates. Cerebral oedema is present in 80% of patients with grade IV encephalopathy. It is best assessed with intracranial pressure monitoring (after CT brain scan to exclude other causes of altered sensorium), and treated as for other causes of raised intracranial pressure.

1. Marrero J, Martinez J, Hyzy R. Advances in critical care hepatology. *Am J Respir Crit Care Med* 2003; 168: 1421-6.

K86 TTFF

Acalculous cholecystitis affects a minority of ICU patients (0.2%), but is associated with a mortality of up to 40%. Biliary stasis and sludging, together with ischaemia of the gallbladder wall, can lead to gangrene, ulceration or gallbladder perforation. Right upper quadrant tenderness and fever are common but non-specific signs. Ultrasound may show a thickened and oedematous gallbladder wall, biliary sludge, mucosal sloughing and pericholecystic fluid. Sensitivity and specificity are only moderate in ICU patients, however. CT has greater diagnostic accuracy. Aggressive management is indicated, with either cholecystectomy or percutaneous cholecystostomy.

1. Streat SJ. Abdominal surgical catastrophies. In: *Oh's Intensive Care Manual*. Bersten AD, Soni N, Eds. Edinburgh: Butterworth-Heinemann, 2003.

K87 FTFF

Fever is common in septic arthritis, but has a sensitivity of only 57%, so its absence is not reassuring. Inflammatory markers are usually raised in septic arthritis (i.e. sensitive), but are non-specific, especially in patients with predisposing conditions such as rheumatoid disease. Clinical examination and plain radiography are of limited benefit in differentiating between the various causes of a monoarthritis. Synovial fluid examination is, therefore, mandatory. A white cell count >25,000/mm³ with >90% neutrophils is strongly predictive of bacterial arthritis and should prompt antibiotic therapy while Gram stain and culture results are awaited. Gram stain is at best 50% sensitive (10% for gonococcal arthritis), and culture may be only 80% sensitive. Non-gonococcal arthritis carries a hospital mortality of 7-15% and causes rapid joint destruction; a high index of clinical suspicion is therefore required when interpreting clinical investigations.

1.   Margaretten ME, Kohwles J, Moore D, *et al.* Does this adult patient have septic arthritis? *JAMA* 2007; 297(13): 1478-88.

K88 TTFT

The RIFLE criteria (Table 2) were drawn up in an attempt to standardise definitions of renal failure thus allowing treatments and studies of such patients to be more readily compared. R=risk of kidney injury, I=injury, F=failure, L=loss of kidney function, E=end-stage kidney disease. The first three can be defined by either urine output or serum creatinine criteria. Criteria for risk (elevation of creatinine >1.5X normal or urine output <0.5ml/kg/h for 6 hours or a fall in glomerular filtration rate [GFR] >25%) are sensitive but non-specific, while criteria for failure are more specific but less sensitive in detecting early and more subtle loss of function. It is accepted that while serum creatinine is not an ideal guide to the degree of renal impairment, it is universally measured as part of routine blood testing while GFR is not.

Table 2. RIFLE criteria. *Adapted from Bellomo, et al. Critical Care 2004; 8: R204-12.*

	GFR decrease	Serum creatinine (increase from baseline)	Urine output
Risk	>25%	X1.5	<0.5ml/kg/h for >6h
Injury	>50%	X2	<0.5ml/kg/h for >12h
Failure	>75%	X3	<0.3ml/kg/h for >24h or anuria >12h
Loss	Persistent acute renal failure >4 weeks		
ESKD	End-stage kidney disease (>3 months)		

1. Bellomo R, *et al* and the ADQI workgroup. Acute renal failure - definition, outcome measures, animal models, fluid therapy and information technology needs: the Second International Consensus Conference of the Acute Dialysis Quality Initiative (ADQI) Group. *Crit Care* 2004; 8: R204-12.

K89   TFFT

Midazolam is mainly metabolised by the cytochrome P4503A4 isoenzyme in hepatocytes. Since it has a high intrinsic clearance, its metabolism is considered to be flow-dependent [1]. However, in advanced cirrhosis it accumulates and should be given in a reduced dose [2, 3]. This may be in part explained by reduced liver blood flow through the cirrhotic liver. Remifentanil is an ultra-short-acting opiate which is metabolised by plasma esterases. Its pharmacokinetics are independent of liver function. Atracurium is inactivated both by Hofmann elimination (a non-enzymatic process which occurs at physiological pH and temperature) and by ester hydrolysis (catalysed by non-specific plasma esterases). It can be dosed as normal even in the presence of severe hepatic impairment. Propofol is conjugated in the liver with glucuronides and sulphates before excretion in the urine and requires a lower dose in hepatic impairment.

1. Shelly MP, *et al.* Failure of critically ill patients to metabolise midazolam. *Anaesthesia* 1987; 42(6): 619-26.
2. Pentikainen PJ, *et al.* Pharmacokinetics of midazolam following intravenous and oral administration in patients with chronic liver disease and in healthy subjects. *J Clin Pharmacol* 1989; 29: 272-7.
3. Trouvin JH, *et al.* Pharmacokinetics of midazolam in anaesthetized cirrhotic patients. *Br J Anaesth* 1988; 60: 762-7.

K90   TTFF

A drug with low protein binding has a high free fraction in the plasma; it is the free fraction that is cleared during renal replacement therapy. A drug with a large volume of distribution will have only a small fraction eliminated even if clearance is high. For example, if a clearance of 60L is achieved in a dialysis session for a drug with a volume of distribution of 50L/kg, this represents only 1.6% of the total drug removed for a 75kg patient (total volume of distribution of 3750L). If a drug has a high non-renal clearance, then even efficient renal replacement will be largely irrelevant to its elimination. In dialysis small molecules diffuse more quickly than large ones, so a drug with a low molecular weight will be cleared to a greater extent especially if high flow rates are used (with slower flow rates more time is available for diffusion equilibrium to occur and the difference is less marked).

1. Bohler J, Donauer J, Keller F. Pharmacokinetic principles during continuous renal replacement therapy: drugs and dosage. *Kidney Int* 1999; 56: S24-8.

K91   TFTF

3,4-methylene-dioxymethamphetamine (MDMA) is an amphetamine which causes toxicity by excessive central nervous system stimulation. Peripheral release of catecholamines, inhibition of reuptake of catecholamines and monoamine oxidase inhibition are all features. Excessive activity coupled with disordered thermoregulation may lead to rhabdomyolysis, renal failure and coagulopathy. Hyponatraemia may result from excessive sodium loss in sweat, excessive water intake and enhanced antidiuretic hormone release; hypernatraemia is rare, as is non-cardiogenic pulmonary oedema. Other complications include hypertension, tachyarrhythmias and, rarely, stroke (haemorrhagic or thrombotic) and hepatotoxicity.

1. Mokhlesi B, *et al*. Street drug abuse leading to critical illness. *Intensive Care Med* 2004; 30: 1526-36.

K92   TFFF

The UK Confidential Enquiry into Maternal and Child Health (CEMACH) conducts a triennial enquiry into obstetric mortality and morbidity. Deaths are classified as direct if they result from pregnancy-specific complications (e.g. haemorrhage), or indirect if they result from pre-existing or new disease aggravated by pregnancy. Based on the latest report, the commonest single cause of maternal death in the UK is cardiac disease exacerbated by pregnancy (an indirect cause). The commonest direct cause of death is thromboembolic disease, followed by hypertensive disease of pregnancy and then haemorrhage. Indirect causes outnumber direct causes in the UK by a small margin. Worldwide, direct deaths are far more common, and haemorrhage is the leading cause. Psychiatric disease is the second most common indirect cause of death following cardiac causes. There were six deaths directly attributed to anaesthesia in the latest report (out of a total of 132 direct deaths). A further 31 deaths were contributed to by substandard anaesthetic care. Only one death was as a result of failed intubation. A recurrent theme was the delay in recognition of the seriously ill obstetric patient with subsequent morbidity and mortality.

1. Confidential Enquiry into Maternal and Child Health. Saving mothers' lives: reviewing maternal deaths to make motherhood safer - 2003-2005. London: CEMACH, 2007.

K93   TTFF

Labetalol is an alpha-1 and beta-blocker which decreases systemic vascular resistance, lowers heart rate and reduces myocardial oxygen consumption. It is the mainstay of treatment of hypertension in pregnancy. Hydralazine is an arterial vasodilator which may cause a reflex tachycardia but is an effective antihypertensive in pre-eclampsia where the primary problem is a high systemic vascular resistance. Sodium nitroprusside is a potent arterial and venodilator which should not be instituted without invasive arterial blood pressure monitoring. Onset is rapid (within 30 seconds), and potential side effects include cyanide toxicity, lactic acidosis, profound hypotension and headache; it is not a first-line drug but may occasionally be useful in the treatment of resistant hypertension. Metolazone is a thiazide diuretic which is used for the treatment of chronic hypertension in the community. It is not indicated in the management of pre-eclampsia.

1. Vidaeff AC, Carroll MA, Ramin SM. Acute hypertensive emergencies in pregnancy. *Crit Care Med* 2005; 33(10): S307-12.

K94   FFTF

This patient has clinical and laboratory findings consistent with a normal pregnancy. Alkaline phosphatase levels rise in normal pregnancy, and mild elevation above the non-pregnant normal range should not be interpreted as evidence of cholestasis. Albumin falls due to dilution by increased plasma volume. Total bilirubin is also lowered since albumin is its main carrier protein. The presence of traditional 'stigmata of chronic liver disease' including palmar erythema and spider naevi is common in pregnancy and reflect increased placental oestrogen production. Aminotransferases should be within the normal non-pregnant range, and elevation should prompt a search for a cause.

1. Bacq Y, *et al.* Liver function tests in normal pregnancy: a prospective study of 103 pregnant women and 103 matched controls. *Hepatology* 1996; 23(5): 1030-4.
2. Guntupalli SR, Steingrub J. Hepatic disease and pregnancy: an overview of diagnosis and management. *Crit Care Med* 2005; 33(10): S332-9.

K95   FFTT

Noradrenaline (norepinephrine) is a directly-acting sympathomimetic drug. It exerts most of its effect by α-1 agonism causing an increase in systemic vascular resistance, a reflex vagal bradycardia and fall in cardiac index. It is formed from dopamine through the action of dopamine ß-hydroxylase and is metabolised to adrenaline (epinephrine) by phenylethanolamine-N-methyltransferase in the adrenal medulla. A typical dose range is 0.05-0.5µg/kg/min. It is a coronary vasodilator and increases contractility of the pregnant uterus, which may compromise foetal blood flow and cause foetal bradycardia.

1. Sympathomimetics. In: *Pharmacology for Anaesthesia and Intensive Care*, 2nd Ed. Peck TE, Hill SA, Williams M, Eds. London: Greenwich Medical Media, 2003.

K96   FTTF

Morphine is a lipophilic drug with a half-life of around 2-3 hours and a volume of distribution of around 4L/kg. If a drug is infused it takes about five half-lives to reach a steady state. Doubling the infusion rate will therefore take about 10-15 hours to have full effect; the effect within 30 minutes will be negligible. Clearance, half-life and volume of distribution are related by the formula $t1/2 = 0.693 \times Vd/Cl$ (where Vd = volume of distribution, Cl = clearance, t1/2 = half-life). Therefore, halving the clearance or doubling the volume of distribution (either of which can happen in critical illness) doubles the half-life.

1. Short TG, Hood GC. Pharmacokinetics, pharmacodynamics and drug monitoring in critical illness. In: *Oh's Intensive Care Manual*, 5th Ed. Bersten AD, Soni N, Eds. Edinburgh: Butterworth Heinemann, 2003.

K97   TTTF

Transpulmonary thermodilution requires the delivery of a bolus of 15-20ml of cold fluid (<8°C) through a central venous catheter with temperature-time measurement at an arterial site (usually femoral) with a thermistor-tipped arterial cannula. The temperature-time curve thus produced gives an estimate of cardiac output according to a modified form of the Stewart-Hamilton equation. Further mathematical derivation allows other parameters to be estimated, including extravascular lung water (EVLW) and global end-diastolic volume (GEDV). GEDV is an estimate of preload which may be a better predictor of fluid requirements than central venous pressure. EVLW is a measure of pulmonary oedema together with any inflammatory cellular exudates which may be found in the lungs in acute lung injury (ALI). A normal value is 5-7ml/kg. Serial measurement of EVLW may track the progress of ALI and guide diuretic therapy, and may be a more sensitive marker of pulmonary oedema than chest X-ray. Algorithms guiding fluid management based on EVLW and other parameters exist, but have not been extensively validated. Total intrathoracic blood volume can be estimated by transpulmonary thermodilution, but not total circulating blood volume.

1. Isakow W, Schuster DP. Extravascular lung water measurements and hemodynamic monitoring in the critically ill: bedside alternatives to the pulmonary artery catheter. *Am J Physiol Lung Cell Mol Physiol* 2006; 291: L1118-31.

K98   TTFF

The Waterlow score is extensively validated in a ward setting and predicts pressure sore development. The higher the score the greater the likelihood of a pressure ulcer developing. Patients scoring over 20 are considered at very high risk, while problems are rare with a score of less than 10. This score takes into account several risk factors including incontinence, weight, skin state and patient age. Several other prediction scores exist which tend to be sensitive but not specific. Nursing workload has been shown to increase by 50% if a pressure ulcer is present, since dressing changes and positioning manoeuvres are time-consuming. Pressure ulcers are associated with a huge increase in the risk of death. In a prospective ICU series, mortality was 63% in patients with an ulcer compared with 15% for those without [1]. Patients should be repositioned every 2-3 hours to prevent development of a pressure ulcer.

1. Clough NA The cost of pressure area management in an intensive care unit. *J Wound Care* 1994; 3: 33-5.

2. Keller BPJA, *et al.* Pressure ulcers in intensive care patients: a review of risks and prevention. *Intensive Care Med* 2002; 28: 1379-88.

K99   FFTT

In a study examining the reasons behind critical incidents in the ICU, the authors found that out of 2677 incidents, 50% could be attributed to some form of non-technical skill deficit. A root cause analysis involves detailed examination of all the technical and non-technical factors associated with an adverse incident, including both local and organisational factors. It is extremely time consuming and should be reserved for serious critical incidents. The use of simulators and simulated critical incidents can be a useful means of assessing both the technical and non-technical skills of members of the clinical team; these include communication, clinical vigilance, appropriate prioritisation of tasks, and team working. However, there is potential for participant behaviour to be altered by the presence of a researcher. Attitudinal studies often suggest that ICU staff are aware of the factors contributing to adverse incidents and how to prevent them. However, this may not reflect real life performance; nurses may recognise the need to question a doctor's decision in a survey, but are sometimes reluctant to question such behaviour in real life.

1.   Reader T. Non-technical skills in the intensive care unit. *Br J Anaesth* 2006; 96(5): 551-9.

K100   FTFF

Tracheal stenosis is a common complication of tracheostomy. It may occur in 31% of patients following a tracheostomy, but is clinically significant in only 3-12% of patients. The commonest sites of stenosis are at the level of the stoma, and cephalad to this in the subglottic region. Distal stenosis is less common, but may occur due to ischaemia caused by compression of the tracheal wall by the cuff or tip of the tracheal tube. Patients may present with failure to wean from mechanical ventilation. Alternatively, exertional dyspnoea and failure to cough up secretions effectively may be presenting complaints. Stridor is a late sign, and signifies advanced stenosis (<5-10mm airway diameter). The majority of patients present within 2 months, although late presentation several years after the tracheostomy is well recognised. Tracheomalacia is a very rare complication of tracheostomy.

1.   Epstein SK. Late complications of tracheostomy. *Respir Care* 2005; 50(4): 542-9.

Paper 2

Type 'A' questions

A1 A 26-year-old psychiatric nurse presents with nausea, lethargy and fits. She is on no medication and is previously well. She is post-ictal with a GCS of 11 when you assess her. Routine bloods reveal a plasma sodium concentration of 113mmol/L. Which one of the following statements is TRUE:

a. Urinary sodium concentration will be >20mmol/l.
b. Conn's syndrome is part of the differential diagnosis.
c. If due to psychogenic polydipsia then fluid restriction will be sufficient treatment.
d. A water deprivation test is indicated.
e. SIADH may cause this picture.

A2 A 44-year-old homeless alcoholic presents for detoxification in a generally debilitated state. After 4 days in hospital he is admitted to the high dependency area with progressive respiratory failure, tachycardia, diarrhoea, ataxia and progressive renal impairment. Blood tests show sodium 133mmol/L, potassium 5.1mmol/L, urea 14mmol/L (39mg/dL), creatinine 244µmol/L (2.76mg/dL), albumin 28g/L, phosphate 0.22mmol/L (0.68mg/dL), creatine kinase 2500U/L. Chest X-ray shows upper lobe diversion consistent with mild pulmonary oedema. The MOST LIKELY unifying diagnosis is:

a. Silent myocardial infarction.
b. Wernicke's encephalopathy.
c. Gastroenteritis.
d. Rhabdomyolysis.
e. Refeeding syndrome.

A3   A 65-year-old lady has an anterior myocardial infarction and develops complete heart block with a ventricular rate of 35bpm. She remains alert (GCS 15) and has a blood pressure of 135/82mmHg. Which statement is FALSE?

a.   Transvenous pacing is indicated.
b.   This rhythm is unlikely to resolve over the next few weeks.
c.   Atropine is likely to be useful as a temporising measure.
d.   The level of the block is probably below the atrioventricular node.
e.   Isoprenaline may be useful as a temporising measure.

A4   The following are true of outcomes following cardiac arrest EXCEPT:

a.   There is level 1 evidence that tight glycaemic control improves outcome.
b.   Survival to hospital discharge is approximately 8% following out-of-hospital arrest.
c.   Patients having peri-operative cardiac arrest have a much better prognosis than other in-hospital cardiac arrests.
d.   Absence of a pupillary light reflex 24h post-arrest predicts poor neurological outcome with high specificity.
e.   The lower the pH in the first 24h post-arrest the higher the mortality.

A5   Regarding acute traumatic cardiac tamponade the following are true EXCEPT:

a.   It is more common in penetrating than blunt trauma.
b.   The jugular venous pressure may be normal.
c.   A fall of >10mmHg in systolic BP during inspiration defines pulsus paradoxus.
d.   An enlarged cardiac silhouette is seen on the chest X-ray.
e.   ECG findings of electrical alternans is pathognomonic of cardiac tamponade.

A6   Regarding the fluid resuscitation of the trauma patient which statement is FALSE?

a.   Resuscitation with large volumes of crystalloid increases the incidence of abdominal compartment syndrome.
b.   Hypertonic saline has been shown to increase survival compared with crystalloid.
c.   Arterial base deficit is a better indicator of adequacy of fluid resuscitation than urine output.
d.   Serum lactate is a better indicator of adequacy of fluid resuscitation than urine output.
e.   Rate of clearance of base deficit is correlated with survival.

A7   A 45-year-old man with diffuse axonal injury and a GCS of 7 on presentation has been sedated and ventilated on your ICU for the past 24h. He has no other injuries of note. Intracranial pressure monitoring has not been instituted. Which ONE of the following statements is TRUE?

a.   Positive end-expiratory pressure (PEEP) is contraindicated.
b. $PaCO_2$ should be maintained at 4-4.5kPa.
c.   Thiopentone is the sedative agent of choice.
d.   Plasma osmolality should be kept below 320mosm/L.
e.   Mean arterial pressure should not exceed 90mmHg.

A8   Which of the following features is NOT typical of the neuroleptic malignant syndrome?

a.   Tachycardia.
b.   Hyperthermia.
c.   Autonomic instability.
d.   Extrapyramidal features.
e.   Rapid onset over a few hours.

A9 The following ECG suggests:

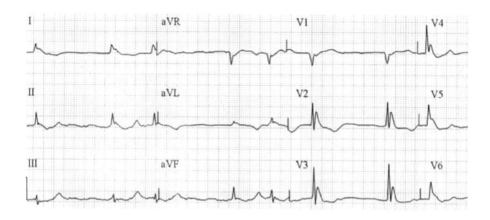

a. Wolff-Parkinson-White syndrome.
b. Hyperkalaemia.
c. Left bundle branch block.
d. Pericarditis.
e. Hypothermia.

A10 Which statement regarding transfusion-related acute lung injury (TRALI) is TRUE?

a. Volume overload is the principal problem.
b. Mortality ranges from 5-25%.
c. It is an immunological diagnosis.
d. It is IgE mediated.
e. TRALI is physiologically distinct from acute lung injury.

A11 A previously well 45-year-old man is assaulted with a baseball bat and sustains a left-sided subdural haematoma (SDH). On arrival in the Emergency Room his GCS is 5, and he undergoes an emergency craniotomy. Following evacuation of the haematoma he is transferred to the ICU. 12 hours later he has a brief tonic-clonic seizure which self-terminates. Which statement is FALSE?

a. SDH carries an increased risk of seizures compared with diffuse axonal injury.
b. Prophylactic phenytoin is effective in preventing early (<7 days) post-traumatic seizures (PTS).
c. Prophylactic anticonvulsants do not reduce the incidence of late (>7 days) PTS.
d. Prophylactic anticonvulsants improve outcome following traumatic brain injury.
e. It is reasonable to start this patient on phenytoin.

A12 Regarding the administration of recombinant factor VIIa which ONE of the following options is TRUE:

a. Its use is associated with a 1-2% incidence of thromboembolic complications.
b. It has a half-life of 12-15 hours.
c. It is given in physiological doses for the management of major haemorrhage.
d. It is licensed for the treatment of major obstetric haemorrhage refractory to surgical management.
e. Disseminated intravascular coagulation is a common complication of treatment.

A13 Regarding nutrition of the patient with major burns which ONE of the following options is FALSE?

a. Aggressive high calorie feeding (>200% of resting requirement) reduces mortality.
b. Enteral feeding is preferred to parenteral.
c. Protein requirement is 1.5-2g/kg/day.
d. Nutritional supplementation with glutamine is of no proven benefit.
e. Hyperglycaemia should be treated aggressively.

A14 Regarding thyroid hormone the following are true statements EXCEPT:

a. Thyroxine (T4) is 90% bound to plasma proteins.
b. Tri-iodothyronine (T3) has greater biological activity than T4.
c. Dopamine inhibits the secretion of thyrotrophin releasing hormone (TRH).
d. Most T3 is produced by de-iodination of T4 in the periphery.
e. No intravenous preparation of propylthiouracil is available.

A15 Regarding extended spectrum ß-lactamase (ESBL)-producing organisms which one of the following statements is TRUE?

a. Most are still sensitive to ceftriaxone.
b. ESBL is ineffective against carbapenems.
c. Antibiotic sensitivity *in vitro* always indicates a suitable antibiotic choice.
d. ß-lactamase inhibitors are highly effective against ESBL-producers.
e. *Streptococcus pneumoniae* is the commonest ESBL-producing organism.

A16 A 58-year-old man is ventilated on the ICU following a Whipple's pancreatoduodenectomy. He is hypotensive (BP 85/65mmHg) and tachycardic (HR 120bpm). Initial oesophageal Doppler measurements include a flow time corrected (FTc) of 290ms, which rises to 310ms following a 250ml fluid challenge. Which statement is TRUE?

a.   A low FTc invariably means more fluid is required.
b.   This patient has normal cardiac contractility.
c.   FTc is a marker of afterload.
d.   Fluid should be titrated to an FTc of 340ms.
e.   Dobutamine should be started at this point.

A17 Which of the following is the LEAST USEFUL marker of the adequacy of the circulation?

a.   Arterial lactate.
b.   Base deficit.
c.   Central venous oxygen saturation.
d.   Pulmonary artery occlusion pressure.
e.   Venous lactate.

A18 A 55-year-old woman is ventilated on the ICU for hospital-acquired pneumonia following aggressive goal-directed fluid therapy in the Emergency Room. She is sedated with propofol 200mg/hour, but remains agitated. The nurses are keen to start a fentanyl infusion. Her BP is 185/105mmHg and HR is 125bpm (sinus rhythm). Which one of the following statements is TRUE?

a.   Significant pain requiring opiates is unlikely.
b.   Her observations indicate she must be in pain.
c.   Problematic hypotension on starting a fentanyl infusion is unlikely in this patient.
d.   Fentanyl is useful in the ICU because of its very short context-sensitive half-life.
e. μ-2 receptor agonism is desirable from an analgesic perspective.

A19 A 66-year-old man is electively ventilated on the ICU following pancreatoduodenectomy. He has a fall in cardiac output shown by oesophageal Doppler monitoring on the first postoperative day, and the possibility of cardiac ischaemia is considered. The pre-operative resting ECG was normal. No ST changes are visible on lead II. Which one of the following statements is TRUE?

a. Significant coronary artery disease is effectively ruled out by the normal resting ECG.
b. Lead II is a sensitive lead for the detection of myocardial ischaemia.
c. Lead CM5 cannot be obtained with a 3-cable system.
d. ST segment changes have a low positive predictive value for true ischaemia.
e. Inferior ischaemia is best monitored with an oesophageal lead.

A20 Regarding diagnosis of pulmonary embolism (PE) which ONE of the following is TRUE?

a. The $S_1Q_3T_3$ ECG pattern is found in 50% of patients with pulmonary embolism (PE).
b. A low probability V/Q scan effectively rules out a PE.
c. Spiral CT is the gold standard investigation.
d. Spiral CT has a sensitivity of >90% for detecting lobar or segmental PE.
e. Transthoracic echocardiography is sensitive for detection of subsegmental PE.

A21 A 34-year-old woman with acute lymphoblastic leukaemia, inflammatory bowel disease and asthma develops a productive cough on the medical ward. On examination her RR is 18 breaths per minute, HR is 85bpm, oxygen saturation is 97% on 4L/min oxygen by facemask. Laboratory arterial blood gas analysis shows a PaO_2 of 3.7kPa (28 mmHg), and the intensive care team is called. The clinical picture is best explained by:

a.   Carbon monoxide poisoning.
b.   Inadequate heparinisation of the blood gas sample.
c.   Extreme left shift of the oxygen dissociation curve.
d.   Artefact caused by an air bubble in the sample.
e.   Pseudohypoxaemia.

A22 Regarding intracranial pressure monitoring devices the following are true EXCEPT:

a.   An intraventricular catheter is the gold standard.
b.   A Camino bolt cannot be re-zeroed once sited.
c.   Infection rates are low with intraparenchymal strain gauge monitors.
d.   The pressure transducer for an intraventricular catheter should be kept at the height of the right atrium.
e.   Parenchymal intracranial pressure monitoring is more accurate than subdural, extradural and subarachnoid monitoring.

A23 Regarding the critical care management of patients with cystic fibrosis which one of the following is TRUE?

a.   The outcome for respiratory failure requiring mechanical ventilation is poor even in younger patients.
b.   *Burkholderia cepacia* is easily eradicated with intravenous antibiotics.
c.   Clinically significant liver disease is usually present.
d.   Massive haemoptysis in these patients is almost always fatal.
e.   Loperamide prophylaxis is useful to reduce gastrointestinal sodium losses.

A24 Which one of the following drugs is NOT suitable for administration via the endotracheal tube during cardiopulmonary resuscitation?

a. Epinephrine.
b. Sodium bicarbonate.
c. Atropine.
d. Naloxone.
e. Lidocaine.

A25 Which of the following has been shown as a routine measure to reduce the incidence of ventilator-associated pneumonia?

a. Semi-recumbent posture.
b. Regular chest physiotherapy.
c. Closed tracheal suction.
d. Prophylactic antibiotics.
e. Routine endotracheal tube change.

A26 A 58-year-old woman sustains a head injury and is rendered unconscious. A CT scan confirms a diffuse intracerebral haematoma not amenable to neurosurgical operation. Over the next 5 days, despite optimal management, her neurological condition fails to improve. She is maintained on pressure support ventilation, and flexes to painful stimuli only. After discussion with the family it is decided to stop artificial ventilation. This is best described as:

a. Euthanasia.
b. Assisted suicide.
c. Withholding of ventilation.
d. Withdrawal of ventilation.
e. Murder.

A27 A 56-year-old woman with a history of COPD is admitted to hospital with respiratory deterioration. On the medical ward she is tiring despite maximal medical treatment including nebulised salbutamol, intravenous aminophylline and corticosteroids. She has a RR of 30 breaths per minute and is alert. Arterial blood gas analysis shows: pH 7.17, $PaCO_2$ 9.8kPa (67mmHg) and PaO_2 8.4kPa (64mmHg) on 40% oxygen. Mechanical ventilation is being considered. Which of the following statements is FALSE?

a. Ventilated COPD patients have lower ICU survival rates than most other medical ICU patients.

b. Survival is better in the absence of a precipitating cause such as infection.

c. Non-invasive ventilation is appropriate for this patient.

d. $PaCO_2$ is a better predictor of the need for mechanical ventilation than PaO_2.

e. Pre-admission health status is an important determinant of survival.

A28 The flow-volume loop of a 40-year-old man shown below is best described by a diagnosis of:

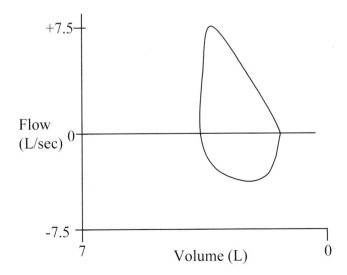

a.   Variable intrathoracic obstruction.
b.   Obstructive airways disease.
c.   Restrictive disease.
d.   Variable extrathoracic obstruction.
e.   Normal spirometry.

A29 The following volume/time graphic on a mechanical ventilator suggests which one of the following?

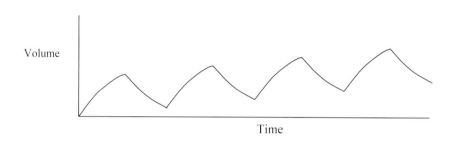

a.   A progressively increasing tidal volume is being delivered.
b.   The set PEEP level has been increased.
c.   The set inflation pressure has been increased.
d.   Functional residual capacity is increasing with each breath.
e.   Dynamic hyperinflation is occurring.

A30 The following are true of the management of atrial fibrillation EXCEPT:

a.   The risk of thromboembolic complications is similar with electrical or chemical cardioversion.
b.   Rhythm control has a proven long-term mortality benefit compared with rate control.
c.   Digoxin is an ineffective rate control agent in the critically ill patient.
d.   Successful cardioversion is more likely in atrial fibrillation of short duration.
e.   Beta-blockers should not be used as first-line therapy in patients with decompensated heart failure.

A31 Which ONE of the following confers the greatest mortality benefit when used appropriately in the management of an acute ST-elevation myocardial infarction (STEMI)?

a. Aspirin.
b. Gylceryl trinitrate.
c. Atenolol.
d. Oxygen.
e. Thrombolysis.

A32 The following waveform is a representation of:

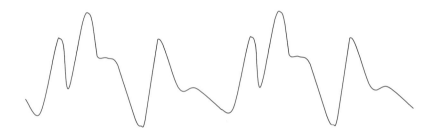

a. The central venous pressure waveform in tricuspid regurgitation.
b. Pulmonary artery pressure waveform in atrial fibrillation.
c. Arterial pressure waveform with intra-aortic balloon counterpulsation.
d. Arterial pressure waveform with premature atrial ectopic beats.
e. ECG recording of torsades de pointes.

A33 Regarding the use of thrombolysis for acute ischaemic stroke which ONE of the following is TRUE?

a. It should not delay the administration of aspirin.
b. It must be administered by endovascular catheter at the site of the occluded artery.
c. A blood pressure of 200/120mmHg is a contraindication.
d. An immediate improvement in neurological status is usually seen.
e. A 'door to needle time' of 30 minutes should not be exceeded.

A34 A patient is referred to the ICU with respiratory failure and bulbar weakness. A diagnosis of myasthenia gravis is under consideration. The following findings would suggest an alternative diagnosis EXCEPT:

a. Raised serum creatinine kinase.
b. Diplopia.
c. A sensory level.
d. An incremental increase in compound muscle action potential with electromyelographic studies.
e. Fasciculations.

A35 A patient with abdominal sepsis develops progressive uraemia and oliguria after 5 days on the ICU. He requires renal replacement therapy, and continuous veno-venous haemofiltration is instituted. The following are appropriate initial settings EXCEPT:

a. Flow rate of 20ml/min.
b. Ultrafiltration rate of 35ml/kg/h.
c. A lactate-buffered replacement fluid.
d. Replacement solution added to blood before passage through the filter.
e. A heparin loading dose of 10U/kg.

A36 Which of the following is the most useful measure in the early management of a patient with rhabdomyolysis following a crush injury?

a. Intravenous crystalloid.
b. Acetazolamide.
c. Mannitol.
d. Sodium bicarbonate.
e. Pentoxyphylline.

A37 The following are major risk factors for the development of stress-related mucosal damage EXCEPT:

a.   Mechanical ventilation.
b.   Diabetes mellitus.
c.   Burns.
d.   Coagulopathy.
e.   Hypotension.

A38 An 85-year-old nursing home resident is admitted to the hospital with a painful, swollen right knee joint. The most appropriate empirical intravenous antibiotic therapy would be:

a.   Flucloxacillin.
b.   Flucloxacillin + gentamicin.
c.   Vancomycin + cefuroxime.
d.   Ceftriaxone.
e.   Clindamycin.

A39 A 44-year-old patient with known oesophageal varices has a massive upper gastrointestinal haemorrhage. Skilled endoscopic assistance is unavailable, and bleeding persists despite appropriate pharmacological therapy. With regard to balloon tamponade with a Sengstaken or Minnesota tube which one of the following statements is TRUE?

a.   Acute bleeding is likely to be successfully controlled.
b.   The tube should be inserted to 30cm before inflation of the gastric balloon.
c.   The gastric balloon is inflated with 50-100ml water.
d.   Maximum traction should not exceed 5kg.
e.   The Sengstaken tube does not have a gastric lumen.

A40 A 55-year-old man is admitted to the ICU with community-acquired pneumonia. He develops multiple organ failure, becomes anuric and requires continuous renal replacement therapy (CRRT). The following patient medications will have significantly increased clearance with CRRT compared with the anuric state EXCEPT:

a. Vancomycin.
b. Gentamicin.
c. Atenolol.
d. Amiodarone.
e. Lithium.

A41 A 22-year-old man is brought to the Emergency Room following ingestion of six 'ecstasy' tablets 8 hours ago. He has been dancing at a nightclub since then, but is now alternately violently agitated and listless. On examination he has a tachycardia (140bpm), and is hypertensive (185/115mmHg). His rectal temperature is 40.3°C. Initial blood tests include a sodium of 114mmol/L (114mEq/L). Appropriate initial measures would include all of the following EXCEPT:

a. Active cooling.
b. Administration of sodium-containing fluid.
c. Arterial blood gas analysis.
d. Gastric lavage to empty the stomach.
e. Intravenous benzodiazepine administration.

A42 Which of the following is NOT one of the criteria to fulfil the standard definition of systemic inflammatory response syndrome (SIRS)?

a. Temperature >38°C or <36°C.
b. Blood pressure <90mmHg systolic.
c. Heart rate >90bpm.
d. Respiratory rate >20breaths/min.
e. $PaCO_2$ <4.3kPa (32mmHg).

A43 A 36-week pregnant woman is admitted to hospital with nausea and vomiting. She is hypertensive (BP 160/100mmHg) but has no headache, visual disturbance or hyperreflexia. Blood test abnormalities include: bilirubin 160μmol/L (9.35mg/dL), aspartate aminotransferase 650IU/L, prothrombin time 24 seconds, fibrinogen 0.5g/L (50mg/dL). Plasma glucose is 2.1mmol/L (38mg/dL). The most likely diagnosis is:

a. Viral hepatitis.
b. HELLP syndrome.
c. Fatty liver of pregnancy.
d. Cholestasis of pregnancy.
e. Ruptured liver haematoma.

A44 Regarding the pharmacology of morphine which of the following statements is TRUE?

a. It undergoes minimal first pass metabolism.
b. It is metabolised to weakly active metabolites in the liver.
c. It inhibits neurotransmission in the central nervous system.
d. Peak effect is reached within 5 minutes of intravenous injection.
e. Respiratory depression manifests mainly as a reduction in tidal volume.

A45 Which one of the following statements regarding amiodarone is FALSE?

a. It is 98% protein-bound.
b. It does not require dose adjustment in renal failure.
c. It has no effect on heart rate if the patient is in sinus rhythm.
d. It has a volume of distribution greater than 2L/kg.
e. It potentiates the effect of warfarin.

A46 Three dose-response curves are plotted on the graph below. Which ONE of the following statements is TRUE?

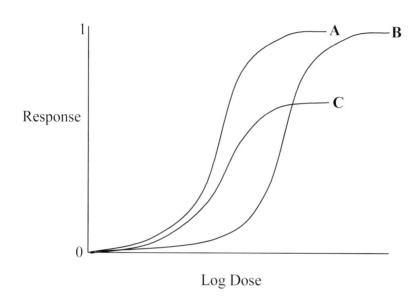

a. If A and B are two drugs acting on the same receptor they have equal efficacy.
b. A is a partial agonist.
c. If A and B are two drugs acting on the same receptor then B is more potent than A.
d. C may represent competitive antagonism of A.
e. A may represent competitive antagonism of B.

A47 The following ventilator graphic is best described by which ONE of the following statements?

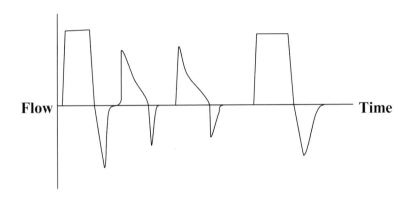

a. Pressure-controlled ventilation with pressure support.
b. Volume-controlled ventilation with pressure support.
c. Significant auto-PEEP.
d. Bronchospasm.
e. Ineffective patient triggering of the ventilator.

A48 The following are true concerning the use of replacement fluids in continuous veno-venous haemofiltration (CVVH) EXCEPT:

a. Bicarbonate-buffered solutions have a short shelf-life.
b. Excessive infusion of lactate-buffered solution may cause metabolic alkalosis.
c. Pre-dilution reduces the risk of filter clotting.
d. Replacement fluids should have a potassium concentration of 1-2mmol/L.
e. Lactate-buffered solutions are usually avoided in liver failure.

A49 A ventilated patient requires transfer to another hospital due to bed shortages in your ICU. Which of the following is NOT a mandatory monitoring requirement during the transfer?

a. Continuous electrocardiography.
b. Pulse oximetry.
c. Central venous pressure measurement.
d. Non-invasive blood pressure measurement.
e. Continuous presence of appropriately trained staff.

A50 A 23-year-old man has been ventilated on the ICU for 3 months following a traumatic brain injury. He has received no sedative medication for the last 5 weeks, and has had a full metabolic screen which is unremarkable. A CT brain scan is unremarkable. On examination, the patient has spontaneous eye opening during waking hours. Cranial nerve reflexes are intact. He shows no recognition of his surroundings. He flexes to painful stimuli (sternal rub) but will not follow a command. He shows no social smiling or apparent recognition of his relatives. His condition is best described as:

a. Persistent vegetative state.
b. Minimally conscious state.
c. Coma.
d. Brainstem dead.
e. Locked-in syndrome.

Paper 2

Type 'K' questions

K51 The following drugs are recognised causes of hypokalaemia:

a. Gentamicin.
b. Triamterene.
c. Piperacillin.
d. Metolazone.

K52 Regarding electrical injury:

a. Skin resistance is 100 times greater when dry than when wet.
b. Ventricular fibrillation occurs at a lower current than asystole.
c. A current of >50mA is required to cause microshock.
d. A current of 1A is sufficient to cause deep burns and neurological injury.

K53 The following are accepted indications for permanent transvenous pacing:

a. Symptomatic second degree heart block.
b. Asymptomatic third degree heart block with documented pauses of >3 seconds.
c. Sinus node dysfunction with documented symptomatic bradycardia.
d. Asymptomatic third degree heart block with a heart rate <40bpm.

K54 A 76-year-old lady is admitted to intensive care following a pulseless electrical activity (PEA) cardiac arrest. She required 28 minutes of cardiopulmonary resuscitation and five doses of IV epinephrine 1mg before regaining spontaneous circulation. On admission to the ICU (pre-sedation) she is comatose with a GCS of 3 and no pupillary reaction to light, but is making spontaneous respiratory effort.

a. Her prognosis would be better if her arrest rhythm were ventricular fibrillation.
b. The length of her resuscitation time before return of spontaneous circulation is not compatible with survival.
c. If she has absent pupillary reflexes at 72h further treatment is futile.
d. Brain swelling on a CT scan accurately predicts poor outcome.

K55 A 28-year-old man receives a stab wound to the upper abdomen. On arrival in the Emergency Room he has a GCS of 15, and is in pain, with a small puncture wound under the left costal margin. BP is 80/40mmHg, HR is 130bpm and RR is 30 breaths per minute. His neck veins are distended. Chest X-ray shows no evidence of pneumothorax or haemothorax. ECG shows right bundle branch block and T wave inversion in lead V1. A focused abdominal ultrasound for trauma (FAST) scan shows the presence of pericardial fluid.

a. Transthoracic echocardiography is the diagnostic technique of choice when considering traumatic cardiac tamponade as a diagnosis.
b. A CT scan of the thorax should be performed immediately to confirm the suspected diagnosis.
c. Rapid fluid infusion should be avoided to prevent right heart failure.
d. Removal of at least 300ml fluid is required to materially improve the clinical condition.

K56 A 34-year-old man is involved in a car accident at high speed. He is the driver and is wearing a seatbelt. He is neurologically intact on arrival in the Emergency Room, but is haemodynamically unstable and has a positive diagnostic peritoneal lavage. He also has bilateral closed femoral fractures. He is taken to the operating theatre for an emergency laparotomy.

a. Definitive surgery must be performed before transfer to the intensive care unit.
b. Surgical stabilisation of the femoral fractures should be deferred until a later date.
c. Hollow viscus injury must be dealt with immediately.
d. The abdomen must be closed to prevent overwhelming sepsis.

K57 Regarding the use of mannitol for the treatment of raised intracranial pressure:

a. A typical dose is 250-500ml of 20% mannitol as an IV bolus.
b. Intravascular volume depletion is a side effect.
c. It increases calculated plasma osmolality.
d. It has a rapid effect.

K58 Immediate management for a patient suspected of having anaphylaxis includes:

a. High-flow oxygen.
b. Intravenous hydrocortisone 100-200mg.
c. Epinephrine 0.5mg IV bolus.
d. Lie the patient flat and raise their legs.

K59 A 64-year-old man presents with crushing central chest pain. An ECG shows 2mm ST elevation in leads II, III and aVf. He is hypotensive, with a BP of 80/50mmHg and the jugular venous pulse is elevated. The lungs are clear to auscultation; ST segment elevation is present in lead V4R.

a. A nitrate infusion should be started to relieve the chest pain.
b. A fluid challenge of 500-1000ml should be given.
c. A posterior myocardial infarction is the likely diagnosis.
d. Thrombolysis is contraindicated.

K60 A 32-year-old woman suffers a liver laceration in a road traffic accident. During laparotomy she bleeds extensively and requires a 15-unit blood transfusion. Postoperatively she is transferred, ventilated, to the ICU where she develops progressively worsening lung compliance and hypoxaemia (PaO_2 9kPa [68mmHg] on 80% inspired oxygen) over the next few hours. Chest X-ray shows widespread fluffy infiltrates; the pulmonary artery occlusion pressure is 15mmHg.

a. The chest X-ray may be consistent with pulmonary oedema.
b. Diuretic therapy is indicated.
c. Corticosteroids are indicated.
d. Sufficient information is available to diagnose transfusion-related acute lung injury (TRALI).

K61 Regarding the cerebral monitoring of patients with traumatic brain injury:

a. Intracranial pressure is a good surrogate measure of cerebral metabolism.
b. A jugular bulb $SjvO_2$ of <50% has prognostic significance.
c. The greater the $SjvO_2$ the better the neurological outcome.
d. A low arterio-jugular oxygen content difference ($AJDO_2$) implies a poor outcome.

K62 Recombinant factor VIIa is licensed for use in the following scenarios:

a. Second-line treatment of bleeding in major blunt trauma.
b. Emergency reversal of the anticoagulant effects of pentasaccarides (e.g. fondaparinux).
c. Prophylaxis against bleeding for procedures in patients with liver disease.
d. Treatment of major obstetric haemorrhage.

K63 Regarding the physiology of the patient with major burns:

a. Cardiac output is increased in the immediate post-burn period.
b. A hypermetabolic state begins in the first 6 hours post-burn.
c. Acidic drugs have an increased free fraction in the plasma.
d. Sensitivity to non-depolarising muscle relaxants is increased.

K64 Regarding methicillin-resistant *Staphylococcus aureus* (MRSA) infection:

a. Around half of all *Staphylococcus aureus* infections are methicillin-resistant.
b. MRSA infection rates are inversely related to nursing staffing levels.
c. MRSA bacteraemia carries about a 15% mortality.
d. Active surveillance culture of patients is an effective means of reducing MRSA infection rates.

K65 Pulmonary artery occlusion pressure (PAOP) overestimates left ventricular end-diastolic pressure in the following conditions:

a. Mitral stenosis.
b. Mitral regurgitation.
c. Massive pulmonary embolism.
d. Catheter tip outside West zone III.

K66 The following are effective methods of predicting an increase in cardiac output in response to a fluid challenge:

a.   Passive leg raising to 10° with oesophageal Doppler monitoring.
b.   Pulmonary artery occlusion pressure.
c.   A large 'swing' on the arterial line trace in a mechanically ventilated patient.
d.   A fall of 3mmHg in central venous pressure during unimpeded inspiration in a spontaneously breathing patient.

K67 A 65-year-old man is brought to hospital having been trapped in a burning building for 1 hour before extrication. On arrival he is ataxic and listless with a GCS of 12. He has a RR of 30 breaths per minute but is haemodynamically stable with no obvious truncal or limb injuries. Arterial blood gas values include: PaO_2 44kPa (334mmHg), $PaCO_2$ 3.5kPa (26.6mmHg), SaO_2 99% and lactate 10.5mmol/L (95mg/dL). Carboxyhaemoglobin level on co-oximetry is 10.4%. He has a brief seizure.

a.   This patient has severe carbon monoxide poisoning.
b.   A normal lactate would rule out cyanide poisoning completely.
c.   Treatment for suspected cyanide toxicity should not be delayed until laboratory blood cyanide levels are available.
d.   Sodium nitroprusside may be appropriate treatment for this man.

K68 The following are accepted indications for administering sedative medication to a mechanically ventilated intensive care patient:

a.   To manage alcohol withdrawal.
b.   To reduce oxygen consumption.
c.   To reduce the long-term incidence of psychological sequalae.
d.   To provide amnesia covering periods of neuromuscular blockade.

K69 A 67-year-old lady with chronic bronchitis and emphysema is ventilated on the ICU and has the following capnograph trace:

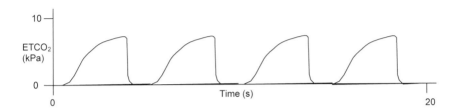

a. The slope of phase II is steeper than normal.
b. The abnormal waveform is explained by late emptying of alveoli with higher V/Q ratios.
c. The end-tidal CO_2 reflects alveoli with the largest time constants.
d. Endobronchial intubation does not produce this picture.

K70 The following are true of thrombolytic therapy for pulmonary embolism:

a. There is a 15% risk of clinically significant bleeding.
b. The $S_1Q_3T_3$ pattern on the ECG is an indication for thrombolysis.
c. Right ventricular function is often improved.
d. Systemic hypotension is an absolute contraindication to thrombolysis.

K71 Regarding delirium in the intensive care patient:

a. It is an independent predictor of increased mortality.
b. It is experienced by 30-40% of mechanically ventilated patients.
c. The Confusion Assessment Method for ICU patients (CAM-ICU) delirium assessment tool can be used in patients unable to communicate verbally.
d. An acute change in mental state is sufficient to make a diagnosis of ICU delirium using the CAM-ICU system.

K72 Concerning Doppler ultrasound:

a. The Doppler effect states that observed frequency increases as the source moves closer to the observer.
b. In colour flow Doppler, a red colour indicates arterial blood flow.
c. For blood flow measurement the probe should ideally be perpendicular to the direction of flow.
d. Blood flow velocity is proportional to the cosine of θ (theta) according to the Doppler equation.

K73 A 44-year-old woman requires ventilation for acute pancreatitis with associated lung injury. On the eighth day of mechanical ventilation she develops new infiltrates on the chest X-ray and a rising white cell count. A diagnosis of ventilator-associated pneumonia (VAP) is made and antibiotics are commenced.

a. The diagnosis should be confirmed microbiologically prior to antibiotic treatment.
b. Tracheobronchial aspiration has a high negative predictive value.
c. Quantitative cultures (e.g. protected specimen brushings) have a high specificity for VAP.
d. Levofloxacin is a suitable antibiotic if empirical treatment is warranted.

K74 Regarding the measurement of lung compliance in mechanically ventilated patients:

a. Static compliance calculation requires knowledge of plateau pressure and PEEP.
b. Dynamic compliance calculation requires knowledge of plateau pressure and PEEP.
c. Static compliance is greater than dynamic compliance for the same patient.
d. Bronchospasm has more effect on dynamic compliance than static.

K75 In a patient with known Wolff-Parkinson-White syndrome who presents with fast atrial fibrillation, appropriate pharmacotherapy includes:

a. Procainamide.
b. Digoxin.
c. Verapamil.
d. Flecainide.

K76 A 72-year-old woman with recent onset fast atrial fibrillation is admitted to the coronary care unit. She complains of severe abdominal pain and looks generally unwell. On examination her abdomen is soft and minimally tender, with no guarding. Arterial blood gas analysis shows profound metabolic acidaemia. Appropriate initial steps include:

a. Obtaining a surgical opinion as this lady may need an urgent laparotomy.
b. Give intravenous morphine and observe overnight while fluid resuscitating.
c. Urgent abdominal ultrasound.
d. Thrombolysis.

K77 The following physiological observations are commonly seen in patients with an acute exacerbation of chronic obstructive pulmonary disease:

a. Reduced respiratory compliance.
b. Increased pulmonary vascular resistance.
c. Increased resistive load.
d. Increased mechanical efficiency of the diaphragm.

K78 A 23-year-old music student presents to the Emergency Room with sudden onset dyspnoea. She has been previously diagnosed with asthma and has a salbutamol inhaler which she has used without effect. There is no history of trauma or foreign body inhalation. On examination, she is unable to talk in sentences, and has a heart rate of 120bpm (sinus tachycardia). Oxygen saturation is 100% on a non-breathing mask with 15L/min oxygen. A flow-volume loop is measured showing the following:

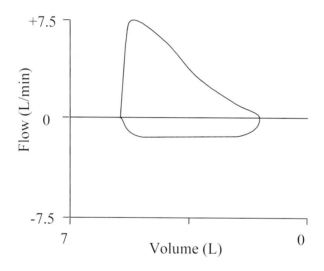

a.   The inspiratory limb of the flow-volume loop is normal.
b.   The flow-volume loop is consistent with bronchospasm.
c.   Steroids and bronchodilators should be administered.
d.   Awake fibreoptic intubation is indicated.

K79 Regarding the use of synchronised DC cardioversion for new onset atrial fibrillation in ICU surgical patients:

a. Sinus rhythm is initially restored in over 95% of cases.
b. Successful DC cardioversion of new onset atrial fibrillation is less likely in medical than surgical patients.
c. Most successfully cardioverted patients maintain sinus rhythm in the first 48 hours.
d. Successful cardioversion is unlikely if the first two shocks are unsuccessful.

K80 The following favour a strategy of primary angioplasty over thrombolysis in patients with an acute ST-elevation myocardial infarction (STEMI):

a. Cardiogenic shock.
b. Late presentation (onset of symptoms >3h ago).
c. 'Door-to-balloon time' likely to exceed 90 minutes.
d. Diagnosis of STEMI in doubt.

K81 A 44-year-old man with dilated cardiomyopathy develops cardiogenic shock while on the waiting list for a heart transplant. His condition is refractory to maximal medical therapy, and placement of a left ventricular assist device (LVAD) is considered.

a. Blood flow produced by an LVAD may be pulsatile or non-pulsatile.
b. The LVAD takes blood from the right ventricle or vena cava and pumps it into the aorta.
c. An LVAD will increase cardiac output much more than intra-aortic balloon counterpulsation.
d. This patient could be maintained on a LVAD for several months.

K82 A 58-year-old man attends the Emergency Room with a dense left hemiparesis which developed suddenly 2 hours ago. BP is 175/105mmHg. A CT brain scan shows no evidence of haemorrhage. Thrombolysis is considered.

a.   Thrombolysis reduces death and dependency rates in carefully selected stroke patients.
b.   Thrombolysis must be given within 12 hours of presentation for the greatest benefit.
c.   Haemorrhagic transformation is not significantly greater with thrombolysis than placebo.
d.   There is no contraindication to thrombolytic therapy from the information given.

K83 A previously well 28-year-old man presents to the Emergency Room with acute confusion. He has been complaining of a headache for the past 2 days. On examination he has a low-grade pyrexia, appears disorientated and has a mild left-sided hemiparesis. There is no history of recent foreign travel. General examination is unremarkable except for the presence of a cold sore.

a.   Lumbar puncture is the initial investigation of choice.
b.   Viral meningitis is the most likely diagnosis.
c.   Empirical acyclovir is mandatory.
d.   CT brain scan is not a useful investigation in this case.

K84 Regarding acute renal failure (ARF) on the ICU:

a.   Hypovolaemia is the commonest predisposing factor in patients with established ARF.
b.   Mortality is not significantly different between ICU patients with and without ARF.
c.   The prevalence of ARF requiring renal replacement therapy in intensive care patients is about 45%.
d.   The vast majority (86%) of ARF survivors are dialysis-independent on hospital discharge.

K85 Regarding stress ulceration in ICU patients:

a. Stress-related mucosal damage usually takes 3-5 days to develop.
b. The incidence of clinically important gastrointestinal bleeding in ICU patients is 1.5%.
c. Bleeding from stress ulcers is associated with significantly increased ICU mortality.
d. Acid suppression is an effective intervention.

K86 A 35-year-old man has been ventilated on the ICU for 6 days following a road traffic accident and emergency laparotomy. He is jaundiced with a bilirubin of 62μmol/L (3.6mg/dL). The following would support a diagnosis of 'ICU jaundice':

a. Dilatation of the biliary tree on ultrasound.
b. Grade III or IV encephalopathy.
c. An aspartate aminotransferase (AST) level of 1500U/L.
d. Intrahepatic cholestasis on liver histology.

K87 The following are common findings in a patient with profound myxoedema:

a. Coma.
b. Hyponatraemia.
c. Elevated creatine kinase.
d. Low/undetectable thyrotrophin.

K88 Regarding the detection of impaired renal function in critically ill patients:

a. The Cockroft-Gault formula requires a urinary creatinine value.
b. A normal serum creatinine measurement indicates normal renal function in critically ill patients.
c. Measurement of the GFR requires a 24-hour urine collection.
d. Calculated GFR correlates well with measured GFR.

K89 Regarding tight glycaemic control in critically ill patients:

a. Maintenance of normoglycaemia is of no benefit in medical ICU patients.
b. Beneficial effects of tight glucose control in surgical patients relate to the dose of insulin used rather than the glucose levels *per se*.
c. Patients with a longer ICU stay (>5 days) benefit the most.
d. Hypoglycaemic episodes are more likely with enteral than with parenteral feeding.

K90 The following are elements of the 6-hour sepsis resuscitation care bundle as advocated by the Surviving Sepsis Campaign group:

a. Serum lactate measurement.
b. Administration of recombinant human activated protein C.
c. Achievement of a central venous oxygen saturation of >70%.
d. Administration of broad spectrum antibiotics within the first 3 hours.

K91 A 46-year-old woman arrives in the Emergency Room with a suspected community-acquired pneumonia. She has a temperature of 38.3°C, a BP of 85/40mmHg, a HR of 105bpm and a RR of 24 breaths per minute. Chest X-ray shows consolidation in the left lower zone, and green sputum is expectorated. Initial blood cultures are negative. Arterial blood gas analysis (on 60% oxygen via high-flow mask) shows: pH 7.32, $PaCO_2$ 3.8kPa (28.9mmHg), PaO_2 8.9kPa (67.6mmHg), base excess -7.3mmol/L and lactate 3.4mmol/L (30mg/dL). A fluid challenge is given.

a. The systemic inflammatory response syndrome (SIRS) is present.
b. Sepsis cannot be diagnosed without a positive blood culture.
c. Severe sepsis is present.
d. Septic shock is present.

K92 Regarding the use of high-frequency oscillatory ventilation (HFOV) in adult patients with the acute respiratory distress syndrome (ARDS) compared with conventional mechanical ventilation:

a. Mean airway pressure is usually higher.
b. Early improvement in oxygenation is typical.
c. Mortality is significantly reduced in surgical patients.
d. Less arterial CO_2 is eliminated.

K93 Regarding amniotic fluid embolism:

a. Hypoxia is most commonly due to bronchospasm.
b. The diagnosis should be questioned in the absence of hypotension.
c. Disseminated intravascular coagulation occurs in 5-10% of patients.
d. The majority of survivors have a permanent neurological deficit.

K94 Regarding the pharmacology of non-steroidal anti-inflammatory drugs (NSAIDs):

a. Bronchospasm may be precipitated by increased bradykinin production.
b. Reduced thromboxane A_2 synthesis reduces platelet aggregation.
c. NSAIDs are excreted unchanged in the urine.
d. NSAIDs have low protein binding and a high volume of distribution.

K95 Regarding amiodarone toxicity:

a. Corneal microdeposits are rare.
b. Pulmonary toxicity does not occur with short-term therapy.
c. Elevation of hepatic transaminases is common.
d. Neurotoxicity is a dose-related problem.

K96 The following graph illustrates the decline in plasma concentration of a drug over time. The curve of this line can be described by the following equation: $C = C_0 e^{-kt}$.

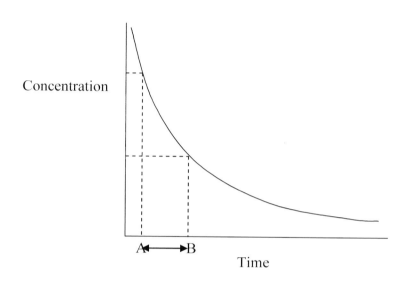

a.   This is an example of first order kinetics.
b.   A two compartment model is shown.
c.   The time constant is the difference between points A and B.
d.   K is the elimination rate constant.

K97 Regarding the use of lithium dilution to measure cardiac output in the ICU:

a.   It cannot be used in patients taking lithium carbonate.
b.   It cannot be used in patients who have previously received atracurium.
c.   Anaemia affects the measurement.
d.   Central venous access is not required.

K98 A patient on the ICU develops acute renal failure and is commenced on haemofiltration. The following measures will increase the efficiency of solute clearance:

a. Increasing blood flow rate.
b. Pre-dilution instead of post-dilution.
c. Increasing the surface area of the filter.
d. Using arteriovenous rather than venovenous renal replacement.

K99 The following factors are associated with a greater likelihood of a critical incident occurring during a patient's care on the ICU:

a. High severity of illness.
b. Long stay.
c. Higher level of care.
d. Renal replacement therapy.

K100 A 35-year-old woman has been ventilated on your ICU for 3 months following an insulin overdose. She has had no sedation for the last month but shows no interaction or apparent awareness despite periods of eye opening. A CT brain scan and metabolic screening show no reversible features. A diagnosis of persistent vegetative state is considered. The following features would rule out this diagnosis:

a. Intact sleep-wake cycle.
b. Bowel and bladder incontinence.
c. Spontaneous movements.
d. Social smiling.

Paper 2

Type 'A' answers

A1   E

The differential diagnosis of hyponatraemia is broad and includes syndrome of inappropriate antidiuretic hormone secretion (SIADH), drugs, GI tract losses, adrenocortical failure, diuretic therapy, renal, cardiac and hepatic failure and psychogenic polydipsia. A low plasma sodium value may be accompanied by a low or high urinary sodium value. A water deprivation test can help distinguish between diabetes insipidus and psychogenic polydipsia, but sodium of 113mmol/L on presentation effectively excludes the former which is a failure to reabsorb free water in the collecting ducts causing a very dilute diuresis and consequent hypernatraemia. Conn's syndrome (primary hyperaldosteronism) is characterised by renal sodium and water retention and causes hypertension but not hyponatraemia. Nephrogenic diabetes insipidus may cause high plasma osmolality and sodium, and inappropriately dilute urine. Regardless of the cause this requires aggressive treatment to increase plasma sodium in a controlled fashion; this may include the judicious use of diuretics and hypertonic saline. A rise of 4-6mmol/L plasma sodium should be enough to prevent fitting, after which fluid restriction and gradual sodium increase may be sufficient.

1.   Adrogue HJ, Madias NE. Hyponatraemia. *New Engl J Med* 2000; 342(21): 1581-9.

A2   E

The refeeding syndrome occurs when a chronically malnourished patient receives re-nutrition. It is characterised by a low serum phosphate with any of a variety of clinical features including arrhythmias and cardiac failure, Wernicke's encephalopathy, leukocyte and platelet dysfunction, rhabdomyolysis, renal failure and myopathy. All abnormalities are secondary to hypophosphataemia, which is a consequence of elevated levels of insulin which are part of the switch from a starvation state to carbohydrate metabolism. It may occur with either enteral or parenteral nutrition. At risk patients should receive a calorie and carbohydrate restricted diet, with daily electrolyte monitoring, prophylactic thiamine and intravenous phosphate replacement if <0.5mmol/L or symptomatic.

1.   Fung AT, Rimmer J. Hypophosphataemia secondary to oral refeeding syndrome in a patient with long-term alcohol misuse. *MJA* 2005; 183(6): 324-6.

A3   C

Third degree heart block is an accepted indication for transvenous pacing even in the absence of symptoms if the heart rate is <40bpm. This rhythm may occur as a consequence of inferior or anterior myocardial infarction (MI). When third degree heart block is seen as a complication of inferior MI, occlusion in the right coronary artery territory affects the atrioventricular (AV) node; this is likely to be temporary. With anterior MI, the occlusion is in a branch of the left anterior descending artery and affects the infranodal conducting system and, therefore, removing vagal tone on the sino-atrial (SA) and AV nodes is unlikely to be helpful. Isoprenaline has a chronotrophic action independent of the AV node, however, and may increase heart rate, but also can precipitate cardiac ischaemia and should be used with caution.

1.   Kaushik V, *et al.* Bradyarrhythmias, temporary and permanent pacing. *Crit Care Med* 2000; 28(10): N121-8.

A4   A

Survival to discharge following out-of-hospital cardiac arrest (OHCA) is 7-10%. After in-hospital cardiac arrest (IHCA) it is 18%, although the subgroup of peri-operative IHCA patients has a 43.9% survival to discharge. The absence of pupillary light reflexes at 24h has been shown to be a specific predictor of poor neurological outcome. The lowest pH in the first 24h post-arrest correlates with mortality when it is below 7.25, presumably reflecting the duration of the arrest and the quality of organ function in the post-resuscitation phase. Although tight glucose control has been shown to improve outcome in surgical ICU patients, this has not been studied prospectively in comatose arrest survivors. However, observational studies indicate that the lowest mortality is associated with a lowest blood glucose concentration of 5-7mmol/L in the first 24h.

1. Nolan JP, *et al.* Outcome following admission to UK intensive care units after cardiac arrest: a secondary analysis of the ICNARC Case Mix Programme Database. *Anaesthesia* 2007; 62: 1207-16.

A5   D

Cardiac tamponade is a rare complication of blunt trauma, but is relatively common in penetrating thoracic or upper abdominal trauma. It is the most common presentation of penetrating cardiac injury. Although the JVP is usually raised it may be low in the presence of associated haemorrhage outside the pericardial sac. In chronic cases of cardiac tamponade enlargement of the cardiac silhouette is usual, but not in acute cases where the low compliance of the pericardium leads to rapid tamponade. Electrical alternans is characterised by alternating levels of ECG voltage of the P wave, QRS complex, and T wave due to the heart swinging with a large effusion. It is a specific but insensitive sign.

1. deCastro MA, Schwartz DE. Pericardial disease (pericarditis and pericardial tamponade). In: *Critical Care Secrets*, 3rd Ed. Parsons PE, Wiener-Kronish JP, Eds. Philadelphia: Hanley & Belfus, 2003: 166-170.

A6   B

A correlation exists between the magnitude of crystalloid resuscitation and the development of the abdominal compartment syndrome. Although the use of hypertonic saline may reduce the chances of this complication, evidence that it improves trauma survival rates compared with standard fluid resuscitation is lacking. Both arterial base deficit and serum lactate are better indicators of the adequacy of volume resuscitation than clinical markers such as blood pressure and urine output. Both initial base deficit and rate of improvement of base deficit are correlated with survival - failure to normalise a base deficit within 2 days of injury is associated with a poor prognosis.

1.   Deitch EA, *et al.* Intensive care unit management of the trauma patient. *Crit Care Med* 2006; 34(9): 2294-301.

A7   D

PEEP may be used especially in hypoxaemic patients, but care should be taken not to use excessive levels, since this could obstruct venous return and increase intracranial pressure (ICP). $PaCO_2$ should be maintained at around 4.5-5kPa; lower levels may cause cerebral artery vasoconstriction and compromise cerebral perfusion. Thiopentone has a high fat solubility and a long elimination half-life, and may be associated with increased risk of nosocomial infections. It is not the first choice sedative although it remains a therapeutic option in cases of refractory raised ICP. A high mean arterial pressure (MAP) may be an appropriate response to raised ICP and should not be treated unless very high in the absence of ICP monitoring, since this may compromise cerebral perfusion pressure (CPP). Administration of mannitol or hypertonic saline are useful therapeutic manoeuvres in cases of raised ICP, but plasma osmolality should be measured and not exceed 320mosm/l, since this is associated with neurological and renal side effects.

1.   Helmy A, Vizcaychipi M, Gupta AK. Traumatic brain injury: intensive care management. *Br J Anaesth* 2007; 99 (1): 32-42.

A8   E

The neuroleptic malignant syndrome is an idiosyncratic reaction to dopamine antagonists including all antipsychotics. It is characterised by autonomic instability, extrapyramidal neurological findings and altered mental state which may range from drowsiness to coma. Onset is typically over a few days. Although dantrolene is often used as part of the management of this condition, its efficacy is questionable.

1. Reulbach U, *et al.* Managing an effective treatment for neuroleptic malignant syndrome. *Crit Care* 2007; 11(1): R4.

A9   E

The ECG is taken from a patient with hypothermia. J waves (Osborn waves) are seen especially in leads V2 to V5. The J wave is a convex positive deflection at the junction of the QRS complex and the ST segment (the J point). It is specific for hypothermia (though not sensitive), and appears at temperatures below 33°C. It represents abnormality in the earliest phase of ventricular repolarisation. While the height of the deflection correlates with the degree of hypothermia, this is of no prognostic value. Other ECG features of hypothermia include atrial fibrillation with slow ventricular response (shown here), a widened QRS complex, and a prolonged QT interval. Wolff-Parkinson-White syndrome is characterised by a short PR interval and a slurring of the upstroke of the QRS complex. Hyperkalaemia is suggested by tall, peaked T waves, a long PR interval or absent P wave, and a broadened QRS complex. Left bundle branch block features a wide QRS complex (>120ms) with an RSR pattern in V6 accompanied by T-wave inversion in the lateral leads. Pericarditis is associated in the acute stage with widespread 'saddle shaped' (concave-upwards) ST elevation across multiple chest leads.

1. Bargout R, Lucas BP. A homeless 63-year-old man with an abnormal electrocardiogram. *Cleveland Clinical Journal of Medicine* 2002; 69: 62-4.
2. Osborn JJ. Experimental hypothermia: respiratory and blood pH changes in relation to cardiac function. *Am J Physiol* 1953; 175: 389-98.

A10   B

It is a clinical diagnosis based on the temporal relationship between transfusion of blood products and the development of acute lung injury (usually developing within 6 hours of transfusion). The same mechanisms of capillary leak and non-cardiogenic pulmonary oedema underpin TRALI and other causes of acute lung injury.

1.   Silliman C, Ambruso DR, Boshkov LK. Transfusion-related acute lung injury. *Blood* 2005; 105: 2266-73.

A11   D

Post-traumatic seizure (PTS) is classified as early (within 7 days of injury) or late (after 7 days). Risk factors for PTS include a GCS <10, subdural, extradural or intracerebral haematoma, depressed skull fracture and penetrating head injury. Both prophylactic phenytoin and valproate effectively reduce the incidence of early PTS, although this has not been shown to improve outcome despite the obvious potential for seizures to cause secondary brain injury. Prophylactic anticonvulsants have not been shown to reduce the incidence of late PTS. Routine seizure prophylaxis is reasonable in high-risk cases but should be stopped after 7 days unless a specific indication for continued therapy exists.

1.   Brain Trauma Foundation; American Association of Neurological Surgeons; Congress of Neurological Surgeons; Joint Section on Neurotrauma and Critical Care, AANS/CNS. Guidelines for the management of severe traumatic brain injury. XIII. Antiseizure Prophylaxis. *J Neurotrauma* 2007; 24 Suppl 1: S65-70.

A12   A

The incidence of thromboembolic problems in patients treated with rFVIIa is 1% in haemophiliacs, and 1.4% in cases of non-haemophilia coagulopathy. It has a short half-life; the duration of action is 2-3 hours so repeat dosing may be required. It is given in large, supra-physiological doses for major haemorrhage (an off-label indication). A suggested regimen is 200µg/kg followed by 100µg/kg at 1 and 3 hours after the first dose. Licensed indications for rFVIIa are prophylaxis and treatment of bleeding in patients with haemophilia A or B and inhibitory antibodies, or acquired factor VII deficiency. Disseminated intravascular coagulation is rare as a consequence of rFVIIa treatment.

1. Levi M, Peters M, Buller HR. Efficacy and safety of recombinant factor VIIa for treatment of severe bleeding: a systematic review. *Crit Care Med* 2005; 33(4): 883-90.

A13   A

Aggressive high calorie feeding has been shown to increase mortality. Calorie intake over ~40% above resting energy expenditure does not increase lean body mass and increases complications such as fatty liver. Enteral feeding is preferable in the presence of a functioning GI tract, but if absorption is insufficient this may need to be supplemented with parenteral feed. Burns patients have an increased rate of oxidation of amino acids and require a high protein intake (1.5-2g/kg/day). Immunonutrition with supplements such as arginine and glutamine has not been shown to be of benefit in burns patients.

1. Ipaktchi K, Arbabi S. Advances in burn critical care. *Crit Care Med* 2006; 34(9): S239-44.
2. Schulman AS, Willcutts KF, Claridge JA, *et al.* Does the addition of glutamine to enteral feeds affect patient mortality? *Crit Care Med* 2005; 33(11): 2501-6.

A14   A

T4 is 99.97% protein-bound, T3 99.7%. T4 is produced exclusively in the thyroid gland, but most T3 is produced by peripheral deiodination of T4. This process is reduced in critical illness, fasting, malnutrition and by drugs including propylthiouracil, corticosteroids, propranolol and amiodarone. T3 has greater biological activity. Dopamine and somatostatin both inhibit TRH release, as do high circulating concentrations of thyroid hormone. Propylthiouracil exists only in enteral form.

1. Vedig AE. Thyroid emergencies. In: *Oh's Intensive Care Manual*, 5th Ed. Bersten AD, Soni N, Eds. Edinburgh: Butterworth-Heinemann, 2003.

A15 B

Extended spectrum ß-lactamase (of which there are many isoforms) is capable of hydrolysing the majority of ß-lactam antibiotics, including all third generation cephalosporins. ESBL is ineffective against carbapenems, which are the treatment of choice for ESBL-producing organisms. However, ESBL producers may also develop resistance to carbapenems by other mechanisms. In many cases an ESBL-producing organism proves resistant *in vivo* to treatment with an antibiotic (especially cephalosporins) to which it was susceptible *in vitro*. Although ß-lactam/ß-lactamase inhibitor combinations such as piperacillin/tazobactam may be effective *in vitro*, they are often less effective *in vivo*, and should not be used as monotherapy for serious infections. ESBL producers are gram-negative bacilli, of which *Klebsiella pneumoniae* is the commonest.

1. Sturenburg E, Mack D. Extended-spectrum ß-lactamases: implications for the clinical microbiology laboratory, therapy, and infection control. *Journal of Infection* 2003; 47: 273-95.

A16 C

FTc is a marker of afterload (a low FTc indicates a high afterload). Since hypovolaemia causes an increase in systemic vascular resistance, FTc is also an indirect marker of preload and is often used for this purpose. However, other conditions such as hypothermia, cardiac failure and vasopressor therapy may similarly increase afterload (reducing FTc) despite adequate or excessive preload. Although an FTc of ~340ms is considered 'normal', this should not be a target of fluid therapy. As with all forms of cardiac output monitoring, trends are more important than absolute values. If a fluid bolus produces an increase in FTc and a significant (>10%) increase in stroke volume, this suggests that more volume is required. If there is little change, giving further fluid may be harmful. FTc gives no information regarding cardiac contractility (peak velocity is more useful in this respect).

1. Singer M. The FTc is not an accurate marker of left ventricular preload. *Intensive Care Med* 2006; 32: 1089.

A17 D

Raised lactate (arterial or venous) is a useful marker of tissue underperfusion, and failure of elevated lactate to fall has been correlated with worse outcome in numerous studies. Both mixed and central venous oxygenation indicate inadequate circulation if low (<60-80% for mixed $ScvO_2$). While a low pulmonary artery occlusion pressure may indicate hypovolaemia, it is a poor predictor of the adequacy of circulating volume, and bears little relation to the adequacy of tissue perfusion.

1. Antonelli M, *et al*. Haemodynamic monitoring in shock and implications for management. *Int Care Med* 2007; 33: 575-90.

A18 C

Intensive care patients may experience pain from a variety of sources even in the absence of obvious causes such as trauma or surgery. Tracheal suction, invasive monitoring, prolonged immobility and the presence of an endotracheal tube are all potential causes of significant pain. Although her hypertension and tachycardia are consistent with pain, agitation or vasoactive medication could give rise to the same observations. Hypotension is a problem with opiates when patients have been inadequately fluid-resuscitated, since the sympathetic tone maintaining blood pressure is damped by their administration. This lady has been aggressively fluid-resuscitated and is unlikely to develop significant hypotension as a result of a fentanyl infusion. Although fentanyl has a short offset following a bolus dose, it has a much longer context-sensitive half-life (around 300 minutes after an 8-hour infusion, and a similar offset time to morphine after infusion for 24 hours). Opiate analgesia is mediated mainly through μ-1 receptor agonism. μ-2 receptors mediate respiratory depression, nausea, vomiting, constipation and euphoria. No commercially available μ-1 selective drugs exist.

1. Kress JP, Hall JB. Sedation in the mechanically ventilated patient. *Crit Care Med* 2006; 34(10): 2541-6.

A19   D

A normal resting ECG is no guarantee of normal coronary circulation. In one study of vascular patients, 30% of those with a normal resting 12-lead ECG had >75% stenosis of a major coronary vessel. Lead II is the best lead for monitoring rhythm disturbances since its axis parallels the electrical axis of the heart, giving the best visualisation of the P wave. It is an insensitive detector of ischaemia however. Lead V5 is the most sensitive detector of left ventricular ischaemia (75%, increased to 90% with the addition of V4). This requires formal 12-lead monitoring, but most cardiac monitors use a three- or five-lead system. CM5 is a more sensitive detector of ischaemia than lead II, detecting around 90% of ST changes due to left ventricular ischaemia. CM5 can be obtained with a three-lead system (right arm lead over manubrium, left arm over V5, left leg anywhere but traditionally clavicle). The positive predictive value of ST segment monitoring is around 35% (although this will vary with the patient population, e.g. higher in vascular patients, lower in young patients). An oesophageal lead is used in the detection of posterior ischaemia.

1.   Edwards ND, Reilly CS. Detection of perioperative myocardial ischaemia. *Br J Anaesth* 1994; 72: 104-15.

A20   D

The $S_1Q_3T_3$ pattern is found in only 20% of patients with pulmonary embolism (PE). Imaging investigations must be interpreted in the light of the pretest probability of PE, which can be determined using scoring systems such as the Revised Geneva Score. V/Q scans are reported as high, intermediate, low probability or normal. While a normal scan reliably excludes a PE, a low probability scan does not and requires further imaging unless the clinical probability is also low. Although pulmonary angiography is the gold standard, spiral CT is highly sensitive for lobar or segmental PE; it may miss subsegmental PE however. Echocardiography is useful in the assessment of the shocked ICU patient in whom PE is being considered as the cause of the haemodynamic disturbance. In such patients, the absence of right ventricular dysfunction or overload virtually excludes the diagnosis. Echocardiography is not sensitive for detecting subsegmental PE however.

1. Torbicki A, Perrier A, Konstantinides S, *et al.* Guidelines on the diagnosis and management of acute pulmonary embolism: the Task Force for the Diagnosis and Management of Acute Pulmonary Embolism of the European Society of Cardiology (ESC). *Eur Heart J* 2008; 29(18): 2276-315.

A21   E

Pseudohypoxaemia or 'leukocyte larceny' is the term given to a spuriously low partial pressure of oxygen (PaO_2) in the arterial blood gas sample of patients with a very high white cell count. This is due to the consumption of dissolved oxygen in the sample by the metabolically active leukoblasts. Immediate analysis of a sample placed on ice will give a higher and more representative PaO_2. Carbon monoxide poisoning does not lower PaO_2 and is not suggested by the history. Heparin is added to the blood gas sample to reduce protein deposition on the pH electrode used in the blood gas analyser, as well as to prevent clotting in transit. Inadequate heparinisation will not affect the PaO_2 however. Even a significant left shift in the oxyhaemoglobin dissociation curve would be insufficient to achieve 97% oxygen saturation at such a low PaO_2. The presence of an air bubble in the sample has a varying effect on PaO_2 depending on the patient's true value, since the dissolved oxygen in the sample equilibrates with the partial pressure of oxygen in the air bubble (21kPa, 160mmHg). A very hypoxaemic patient would therefore have a falsely elevated PaO_2, whereas a hyperoxic patient would have a reduced PaO_2 which would not fall below 21kPa (160mmHg).

1.   Charoenratanakul S, Loasuthi K. Pseudohypoxaemia in a patient with acute leukaemia. *Thorax* 1997; 52: 394-5.

A22   D

The intraventricular catheter is the gold standard and allows pressure to be transduced with reference to atmospheric pressure by means of a fluid column (as for invasive vascular pressure measurement). The pressure transducer should be kept at the level of the foramen of Munro. This system can be recalibrated as required; cerebrospinal fluid can also be drained to reduce intracranial pressure. Infection is a concern, especially if the intraventricular catheter is in place for >5 days. Strain-gauge devices such as the Camino system can be placed intraparenchymally or intraventricularly, and fibreoptic technology used to transduce pressure. They provide a less damped trace than fluid-filled catheter systems, but cannot be recalibrated once inserted, and are subject to a small amount of drift. Intraparenchymal monitors are more accurate than subdural, subarachnoid or extradural systems, have low infection rates and can be used for extended periods if required.

1. Ross N, Eynon CA. Intracranial pressure monitoring. *Current Anaesthesia & Critical Care* 2005; 16: 255-61.
2. Brain Trauma Foundation, American Association of Neurological Surgeons, Congress of Neurological Surgeons. Guidelines for the management of severe traumatic brain injury. Intracranial pressure monitoring technology. *J Neurotrauma* 2007; 24(Suppl 1): S45-54.

A23   A

The outcome of patients requiring mechanical ventilation for respiratory failure is usually poor. In one UK case series, 5 of 13 admissions survived to discharge, but only two were alive at 6 months. *Burkholderia cepacia* is usually multidrug resistant and extremely difficult to eradicate, but may be sensitive to chloramphenicol, co-trimoxazole or meropenem. Liver disease is common, and is found in 25% when defined by abnormal liver function tests (mildly elevated alkaline phosphatase and γ-glutamyl-transpeptidase levels are common). Clinically significant liver disease is found in only 5%, however, and may cause ascites, oesophageal varices, secondary hyperaldosteronism or coagulopathy. Massive haemoptysis may be precipitated by infection, but outcomes are relatively good in patients who do not require mechanical ventilation; bronchial artery embolisation is an effective treatment. Cystic fibrosis patients are prone to the distal intestinal obstruction syndrome. Care should be taken to maintain good hydration and avoid the use of constipating drugs (including opiates) where possible. Gastrograffin enema, intestinal lavage and rectal N-acetylcysteine are non-surgical treatment options in selected cases.

1. Thomas SR. The pulmonary physician in critical care. Illustrative case 1: Cystic fibrosis. *Thorax* 2003; 58: 357-60.

A24   B

Epinephrine (adrenaline), lidocaine (lignocaine), atropine and naloxone can be given endotracheally if no IV access is obtainable. At least three times the intravenous dose should be given, diluted in 10-20ml of water or normal saline.

1.   Resuscitation Council (UK). *Advanced Life Support*, 5th Ed. London: Resuscitation Council (UK), 2006.

A25   A

Semi-recumbent positioning of ventilated patients has been shown to reduce the incidence of ventilator-associated pneumonia (VAP) in a randomised controlled trial, while the supine position was an independent risk factor for mortality in patients with VAP. There is no good evidence to support the other strategies listed. Hand washing and avoidance of gastric over-distension are other measures recommended by the European Taskforce on ventilator-associated pneumonia.

1.   Ferrer R, Artigas A. Clinical review: non-antibiotic strategies for preventing ventilator-associated pneumonia. *Crit Care* 2002, 6: 45-51.

A26   D

Since the treatment has already been started, D is the correct term. In this case the treatment (artificial ventilation) can be considered both futile and burdensome for the patient, and may therefore be withheld, even if death may be hastened in doing so (the 'doctrine of double effect'). If the primary aim of the doctor withholding this treatment were to hasten the death of the patient, however, this might constitute euthanasia and would be considered unlawful in the United Kingdom and most other countries. 'Assisted suicide' would require the patient's own ideation which is not present. In the UK, the General Medical Council issues guidance regarding end of life decisions.

1. General Medical Council. Withholding and withdrawing life-prolonging treatments: good practice in decision-making. General Medical Council (UK), 2008.

A27   A

Survival depends on many factors including the presence of comorbidities, previous lung function and pre-admission health status. Overall, short-term survival rates for ventilated COPD patients are 63-86%, which is better than most other categories of unplanned medical admissions. Surprisingly, survival following mechanical ventilation in COPD is better in the absence of a major precipitating cause such as pneumonia. This may be explained by the fact that patients with such a cause may require protracted periods of ventilation which expose them to other complications. $PaCO_2$ and pH are better predictors of the need for mechanical ventilation than PaO_2, although they are insufficiently sensitive and specific to allow accurate prediction on an individual basis. Non-invasive ventilation has a superior outcome in this group of patients and is appropriate in the absence of contraindications such as a low GCS, excessive secretions, or cardiovascular instability.

1. Davidson AC. The pulmonary physician in critical care 11: critical care management of respiratory failure resulting from COPD. *Thorax* 2002; 57: 1079-84.

A28   C

The expiratory flow rate and shape of the loop are essentially normal but the vital capacity is greatly reduced. In the flow-volume loop shown it is about 3.5L, whereas the normal value for a man of this age should be around 6L. A variable intrathoracic obstruction (e.g. tumour in the lower trachea) would have a flattened expiratory limb. Obstructive airways disease would have a 'scooped out' appearance to the expiratory limb. A variable extrathoracic obstruction (e.g. laryngeal tumour) would have a flattened inspiratory limb.

1. Respiratory disease. In: *Clinical Medicine*, 4th Ed. Kumar P, Clark M, Eds. WB Saunders: Edinburgh,1998: Chapter 12.

A29 E

The height of each waveform is constant, indicating that a constant tidal volume is being delivered. However, the waveform does not return to baseline on each occasion, and becomes progressively higher. This indicates that not all the gas entering the lungs with each breath is exhaled. Such dynamic hyperinflation is a common occurrence in asthma or chronic obstructive airways disease and can be remedied by increasing the expiratory time. Disconnection of the breathing circuit for a few seconds allows trapped gas to escape returning the waveform to baseline. The functional residual capacity is a property of the patient's lungs and is represented by the baseline of the volume/time curve when gas trapping has been eliminated.

1. Blanch L, *et al.* Measurement of air trapping, intrinsic positive end-expiratory pressure, and dynamic hyperinflation in mechanically ventilated patients. *Respir Care* 2005; 50(1): 110-23.

A30 B

The risk of thromboembolic complications is similar regardless of the mechanism of cardioversion. If atrial fibrillation has been present for >48 hours it should be assumed that thrombus may have formed in the atria and therapeutic anticoagulation should be instituted for 3 weeks before attempting cardioversion if the patient remains haemodynamically stable. Since the atria take some time to return to full function even with the restoration of sinus rhythm ('atrial stunning'), anticoagulation should be maintained for 4 weeks post-cardioversion. Although rhythm control is intuitively a more attractive option than rate control, several large studies have failed to show a long-term mortality benefit over rate control with anticoagulation. In patients with longstanding atrial fibrillation successful cardioversion is unlikely. Although beta-blockers should be used with caution in patients with heart failure, they are not contraindicated in stable patients. In those with decompensated heart failure, however, other agents such as amiodarone have less negative inotropic effect. Digoxin is relatively ineffective in hyperadrenergic states, and is therefore not suitable as monotherapy for the rate control of atrial fibrillation in critically ill patients.

1. Lim HS, *et al.* Clinical review: clinical management of atrial fibrillation - rate control versus rhythm control. *Crit Care* 2004; 8: 271-9.

A31 A

A pooled analysis of 22 trials with over 80,000 patients showed only a small mortality benefit from the use of intravenous or sublingual nitrates (absolute mortality reduction from 7.7% to 7.4%). A mortality benefit from the routine administration of supplemental oxygen or morphine has not been shown. In older trials beta-blockers were shown to confer a modest mortality benefit in STEMI patients who did not receive thrombolysis (absolute reduction ~0.6%), but evidence for a clear mortality benefit is equivocal when administered with thrombolytic therapy in the modern era. Analysis of pooled data from nine trials of fibrinolytic therapy shows an overall relative reduction in 35-day mortality of 18% (from 11.5% to 9.6%). The second International Study of Infarct Survival (ISIS-2) trial showed a relative reduction in the 35-day mortality of 23% (absolute reduction 2.4%) with the administration of aspirin in a dose of 162-325mg. This should be given within 24 hours of STEMI, but has not been shown to be as time-critical as thrombolysis.

1. Antman EM, *et al.* ACC/AHA guidelines for the management of patients with ST-elevation myocardial infarction: a report of the American College of Cardiology/American Heart Association Task Force on Practice Guidelines (Committee to Revise the 1999 Guidelines for the Management of Patients With Acute Myocardial Infarction). *Circulation* 2004; 110; e82-293.

A32 C

The waveform shown is the arterial pressure wave caused by an intra-aortic balloon pump. The cylindrical balloon sits distal to the left subclavian artery and inflates at the start of diastole, gauged by the dicrotic notch on the arterial trace. It remains inflated throughout diastole, the augmented pressure wave increasing coronary perfusion pressure. It deflates during isovolumetric contraction, before ejection of blood from the left ventricle begins. The fall in afterload produced by this deflation reduces cardiac work and oxygen consumption. Typically a modest increase in cardiac output is seen. The waveform shows intra-aortic balloon counterpulsation with a 1:2 ratio.

1. Raper R. Intensive care after cardiac surgery. In: *Oh's Intensive Care Manual*, 5th Ed. Bersten AD, Soni N, Eds. Edinburgh: Butterworth-Heinemann, 2003: 245-53.

A33   C

Aspirin should be given to all ischaemic stroke patients who are not candidates for thrombolysis. The risk of intracranial haemorrhage is significantly increased by thrombolysis, however, and in eligible patients antiplatelet drugs should be avoided. Thrombolysis may be administered by an interventional radiologist directly into the blocked artery, but is more commonly administered peripherally as in ST-elevation myocardial infarction. The consensus upper limits of blood pressure are 185mmHg systolic and 110mmHg diastolic; higher levels may increase the risk of haemorrhagic transformation. Acute reduction of elevated blood pressure in stroke patients risks worsening intracerebral perfusion and should be done with caution if required. The National Institute of Neurological Disorders and Stroke (NINDS) rt-PA study [1] showed no difference in neurological improvement between thrombolysis and control groups at 24 hours, although lower death and dependency rates were shown at 3 months. Thrombolysis should be administered in the first 3 hours following onset of symptoms for maximum benefit.

1. The National Institute of Neurological Disorders and Stroke Study Group. Tissue plasminogen activator for acute ischaemic stroke. *N Engl J Med* 1995; 333(24): 1581-7.
2. Khaja AM, Grotta JC. Established treatments for acute ischaemic stroke. *Lancet* 2007; 369: 319-30.

A34   B

The differential diagnosis of myasthenia gravis (MG) is broad, and in a first presentation other diseases must be ruled out. A raised serum creatine kinase would suggest some form of myopathy. Cervical myelopathy may mimic the motor weakness of MG, and may have a sensory level which suggests spinal cord pathology rather than a neuromuscular junction problem. Fasciculations are characteristic of lower motor neurone pathology and are classically seen in patients with motor neurone disease.

Electromyelography showing an incremental increase in compound muscle action potential response with high rates of repetitive stimulation is in keeping with the Lambert-Eaton myasthenic syndrome. Ocular symptoms are present in 90% of MG patients, including diplopia and ptosis.

1.   Lacomis D. Myasthenic crisis. *Neurocrit Care* 2005; 3: 189-94.

A35   A

A typical flow rate would be 120ml/min; very low flow rates increase the likelihood of the filter clotting and provide inefficient clearance of solutes. Ultrafiltration rates of 35-45ml/kg/h have been shown to improve ICU survival compared with 20ml/kg/h [1]. A lactate-buffered replacement solution is standard, since bicarbonate-buffered solutions have a short shelf life. In cases of hepatic failure, however, the liver is unable to metabolise the lactate to bicarbonate, and in such patients lactate-free solution should be used. The replacement solution can be added to the circuit pre- or post-filter. Some evidence suggests that the former prolongs the life of the filter, at the expense of less efficient clearance of solutes [2]. Various anticoagulation options exist, but heparin is the commonest. A loading dose of 5-15U/kg is usual, followed by an infusion titrated to the measured activated partial thromboplastin time (APTT) of the post-filtration blood to maintain an APTT ratio of 1.5-2. Coagulopathic or uraemic patients may not require additional anticoagulation.

1.   Ronco C, *et al*. Effects of different doses in continuous veno-venous haemofiltration on outcomes of acute renal failure: a prospective randomised trial. *Lancet* 2000; 356 (9223): 26-30
2.   van der Voort PHJ, *et al*. Filter run time in CVVH: pre-versus post-dilution and nadroparin versus regional heparin-protamine anticoagulation. *Blood Purif* 2005; 23: 175-80.

A36   A

Retrospective analysis has shown that vigorous intravenous fluid administration is associated with a reduced incidence of acute renal failure in patients with rhabdomyolysis. While mannitol has several theoretically useful properties in the management of rhabdomyolysis, including a free radical-scavenging action, improved renal blood rheology and a 'flushing out' effect on the renal tubules, it has not been shown to improve outcome compared with fluids alone in a large retrospective study [1]. Bicarbonate or acetazolamide are often given to alkalinise the urine, allowing more (acidic) myoglobin to be dissolved and excreted. However, bicarbonate may have deleterious effects including worsening systemic hypocalcaemia, and has not been shown to confer any benefit over fluid resuscitation alone. Pentoxyphylline is one of several free radical scavengers which have theoretical but largely unproven benefits in the management of this condition.

1. Brown C, et al. Preventing renal failure in patients with rhabdomyolysis: do bicarbonate and mannitol make a difference? J Trauma 2004; 56: 1191-6.
2. Huerta-Aladin AL, Varon J, Marik PE. Bench-to-bedside review: rhabdomyolysis - an overview for clinicians. Crit Care 2005; 9: 158-69.

A37 B

In a prospective survey of ICU patients [1] the two risk factors independently associated with increased risk of clinically significant stress ulcer bleeding were mechanical ventilation for >48h and the presence of a coagulopathy. Several other associations are well recognised, including burns, major trauma, renal failure and hepatic failure. Diabetes mellitus is not a risk factor in this population.

1. Cook DJ, Fuller HD, Guyatt GH et al. Risk factors for gastrointestinal bleeding in critically ill patients. Canadian Critical Care Trials Group. N Engl J Med 1994; 330: 377-81.
2. Stollman N, Metz DC. Pathophysiology and prophylaxis of stress ulcer in intensive care unit patients. Journal of Critical Care 2005; 20: 35-45.

A38 C

In patients with no special risk factors, *S. aureus* and streptococci are the commonest pathogens, and will be covered with flucloxacillin and gentamicin. Patients at risk of MRSA including nursing home residents and recent inpatients should be treated with vancomycin and a second or third generation cephalosporin. Patients at risk of Gram-negative sepsis such as those with recurrent urinary tract infections or recent abdominal surgery should be treated with a second or third generation cephalosporin. The incidence of gonococcal arthritis is falling, and specific cover for this is not required unless clinically indicated by the sexual history or examination findings (skin pustules may be present). Empirical therapy should be started immediately following joint aspiration, and should be guided by local microbiological advice.

1.   Coakley G, *et al*, on behalf of the British Society for Rheumatology Standards, Guidelines and Audit Working Group. BSR & BHPR, BOA, RCGP and BSAC guidelines for management of the hot swollen joint in adults. *Rheumatology* 2006; 45: 1039-41.

A39 A

Acute bleeding is controlled in 90% of cases, although further bleeding is common following balloon deflation (50% of cases). The tube should be inserted to at least 45cm before inflation of the gastric balloon to prevent inflation in the oesophagus. A volume of 300-500ml fluid is required to fully inflate the gastric balloon. Once inflated a pulley system can be used to maintain traction not usually exceeding 1kg. A 250-500ml bag of fluid is an appropriate weight for initial traction. If bleeding continues, the oesophageal balloon may be inflated to the lowest pressure required to stop bleeding (this may be 30mmHg). The oesophageal balloon should be deflated for 5 minutes every hour to prevent mucosal pressure necrosis. Both the Sengstaken and Minnesota tubes have a gastric lumen and two balloons; the Minnesota tube has a fourth lumen for oesophageal aspiration.

1.   Alimentary emergencies. In: *Pocket Consultant: Gastroenterology*, 3rd Ed. Travis SPL, *et al*. Oxford: Blackwell, 2005: 8-15.

A40 D

For a drug to be significantly cleared by renal replacement therapy, it must have low protein binding (only the free fraction is filtered). It must have a low non-renal clearance (otherwise the contribution of the renal replacement to removal of the drug will be irrelevant). It must have a low volume of distribution (Vd) for a significant elimination to occur (haemofiltration may clear 3L/hour of ultrafiltrate, but this is of little importance to the clearance of a drug with a 500L Vd). Amiodarone has a very large Vd, is eliminated in bile and is highly protein-bound and is therefore not significantly eliminated by renal replacement therapy.

1. Bohler J, Donauer J, Keller F. Pharmacokinetic principles during continuous renal replacement therapy: drugs and dosage. *Kidney Int* 1999; 56: S24-8.

A41 D

Active cooling should be initiated if the core temperature exceeds 40°C. Dantrolene has been used for the treatment of hyperthermia in this setting, but its role is unclear and it may cause hepatotoxicity (also a risk of ecstasy poisoning). For mild hyponatraemia simple fluid restriction might be sufficient, but this patient has a very low sodium and is symptomatic. Cautious infusion of normal or hypertonic saline is indicated with careful electrolyte monitoring to avoid rapid increases which could lead to central pontine myelinosis. Gastric lavage is of no use in terms of reducing absorption of the drug unless ingestion occurred within the previous hour, although gastric lavage with ice cold saline would be one option to lower the core temperature. Metabolic acidosis secondary to hypermetabolism or acute renal failure is common and blood gas analysis is an essential investigation. Tachyarrhythmias and agitation may be treated with benzodiazepines or butyrophenones (e.g. haloperidol). Profound hypertension and tachycardia may require a combination of alpha- and beta-blockade; pure beta-blockade is best avoided since unopposed alpha stimulation may cause increased hypertension and cardiovascular collapse.

1. Mokhlesi B, *et al.* Street drug abuse leading to critical illness. *Intensive Care Med* 2004; 30: 1526-36.

A42 B

Standardised definitions of the systemic inflammatory response syndrome (SIRS), sepsis, severe sepsis and septic shock were proposed by the American College of Chest Physicians/Society of Critical Care Medicine consensus conference in 1992. Although non-specific, these provide a framework useful for patient diagnosis, and as a research classification tool. Hypotension does not form part of the criteria for SIRS. An increased minute volume may be suggested by a respiratory rate of >20 breaths/min, or by a respiratory alkalosis.

1. Bone RC, *et al.* Definitions for sepsis and organ failure and guidelines for the use of innovative therapies in sepsis. The ACCP/SCCM Consensus Conference Committee. American College of Chest Physicians/Society of Critical Care Medicine. *Chest* 1992; 101(6): 1644-55.

A43 C

Acute fatty liver of pregnancy (AFLP) is a rare condition with a high mortality (18% maternal, 23% foetal). It occurs in the third trimester and is caused by an enzymatic defect in fatty acid oxidation which causes a microvesicular fatty infiltration of hepatocytes in the absence of significant inflammation or necrosis. It may co-exist with pre-eclampsia, and is characterised by a slowly developing jaundice, elevated transaminases (not usually exceeding 1000IU/L) and derangement of coagulation (elevated prothrombin time, thromboplastin time and decreased fibrinogen). Hypoglycaemia is common, and hepatic encephalopathy may supervene in severe cases. There may be significant clinical overlap with the Haemolysis, Elevated Liver enzymes and Low Platelets (HELLP) syndrome, but marked elevations of bilirubin, hypoglycaemia and severe clotting derangement in AFLP help differentiate the two. Acute right upper quadrant pain and haemodynamic instability would suggest liver haematoma, which could be ruled out by an ultrasound scan. Cholestasis of pregnancy rarely causes a bilirubin level of >100μmol/L (6mg/dL), and does not cause a coagulopathy. Viral hepatitis is always a possibility, but would be associated with higher transaminase levels and does not fit with the clinical history of hypertension in pregnancy.

1. Guntupalli SR, Steingrub J. Hepatic disease and pregnancy: an overview of diagnosis and management. *Crit Care Med* 2005; 33(10): S332-9.

A44   C

Morphine undergoes extensive first pass metabolism such that only 25-30% of an oral dose reaches the systemic circulation. It is metabolised in the liver to morphine 3-glucuronide and morphine 6-glucuronide; the latter has a potency over ten-fold greater than morphine. These metabolites are renally excreted. Morphine acts as a ligand for Gi (inhibitory) proteins on presynaptic nerve terminals in the brain and spinal cord. This causes potassium influx into the neurone, hyperpolarisation and inhibition of neurotransmission. Inhibition of GABA-ergic transmission in this way may 'release the brakes' on descending inhibitory pain pathways in the midbrain among other actions. Peak effect takes 10-30 minutes from the time of intravenous injection. Respiratory depression manifests predominantly as a fall in respiratory rate rather than tidal volume.

1. Analgesics. In: *Pharmacology for Anaesthesia and Intensive Care*, 2nd Ed. Peck TE, Hill SA, Williams M. London: Greenwich Medical Media, 2003: 123-36.

A45   C

Amiodarone is highly protein-bound and has a large volume of distribution (up to 70L/kg). It slows diastolic depolarisation of sinus node 'pacemaker' cells and causes a 15% reduction in heart rate of patients in sinus rhythm. It displaces many drugs from their binding sites on plasma proteins, including digoxin and warfarin. It is metabolised by the liver to an active metabolite, desethylamiodarone, which is excreted in bile; no dose adjustment is required in renal failure.

1. Sasada M, Smith S. *Drugs in Anaesthesia & Intensive Care*, 3rd Ed. New York: Oxford University Press, 2003.

A46   A

A full agonist is able to elicit a maximal response when bound to a receptor system in sufficient concentration (high intrinsic activity or efficacy). Both lines A and B might represent full agonists of equal efficacy. Drug A, however, would be more potent than drug B since it causes maximal response at a lower dose. A partial agonist is a drug which has less than 100% intrinsic activity; even if it has high affinity for the receptor in question it cannot achieve maximal response regardless of dose. C might represent such a drug, but might also represent non-competitive antagonism of drug A. B might represent competitive antagonism of drug A, meaning that antagonism can be overcome and maximal effect achieved by sufficiently increasing the concentration of the agonist.

1. Drug action. In: *Pharmacology for Anaesthesia and Intensive Care*, 2nd Ed. Peck TE, Hill SA, Williams M. London: Greenwich Medical Media, 2003: 29-41.

A47   B

The flow-time graphic can give useful information about the adequacy of mechanical ventilation. In the example shown, the first and last breaths are volume-controlled (with the typical square inspiratory flow waveform). The middle two breaths are pressure-supported with a rapid peak flow achieved to generate the set level of pressure support. Since the expiratory flow reaches zero prior to the next inspiration, there is no evidence of auto-PEEP in the graphic shown. Bronchospasm might be suggested by a long expiratory time during pressure-support ventilation or a failure of expiratory flow to return to baseline prior to the next breath (i.e. evidence of auto-PEEP). Ineffective patient triggering of the ventilator would mean a spontaneous breathing effort not accompanied by a mechanically supported breath. The flow-volume graphic would display an abrupt and transient increase or decrease in flow, depending on whether the patient effort occurred during mechanical inspiration (increase in positive flow) or expiration (decrease in negative flow).

1. Nilsestuen JO, Hargett KD. Using ventilator graphics to identify patient-ventilator asynchrony. *Respir Care* 2005; 50(2): 202-34.
2. Pruitt WC. Ventilator graphics made easy. *Rt: the Journal for Respiratory Care Practitioners* 2002; 15(1): 23-4, 50.

A48 D

Replacement fluids usually contain lactate which is metabolised by the liver to bicarbonate, replacing the endogenous bicarbonate ion that is freely filtered during CVVH (as are all molecules <20kDa molecular weight). Excessive lactate administration may therefore lead to metabolic alkalosis assuming the liver is functioning normally. If there is liver failure the lactate is not metabolised and may accumulate. Pre-dilution (adding replacement fluid prior to passage through the filter) reduces the haematocrit of the filtered blood and may reduce filter clotting, but at the expense of less efficient solute clearance. Replacement fluid should have a normal potassium concentration unless extreme hyperkalaemia is present, since the aim of haemofiltration is to discard plasma containing unwanted solutes (e.g. urea) and replace it with a similar volume of physiologically normal replacement fluid.

1.   Forni LG, Hilton PJ. Continuous hemofiltration in the treatment of acute renal failure. *New Engl J Med* 1997; 336: 1303-9.
2.   Hall NA, Fox AJ. Renal replacement therapies in critical care. *CEACCP* 2006; 6: 197-202.
3.   White SA, Goldhill DR. Is Hartmann's the solution? *Anaesthesia* 1997; 52: 422-7.

A49 C

Minimum standards of monitoring are detailed in guidelines produced by the Intensive Care Society (UK) and the American College of Critical Care Medicine (USA). Patients should be monitored to the same basic standard that would be expected on the ICU. Continuous ECG, pulse oximetry and non-invasive blood pressure measurement are mandatory. Invasive blood pressure measurement is desirable given the unreliability of non-invasive measurement in a moving ambulance, and should be considered in the vast majority of critically ill patients undergoing inter-hospital transfer. Central venous pressure monitoring may be of use in optimising volume status, but is not mandatory. Capnography is also considered by the Intensive Care Society (ICS) to be a minimum standard of monitoring in ventilated patients. Two appropriately trained staff must accompany the patient at all times; the ICS specifies an 'appropriately trained medical practitioner', while the ACCCM specifies a physician or nurse with appropriate training.

1.   Intensive Care Society. Transport of the Critically Ill Adult. London: Intensive Care Society, 2002.
2.   Warren J, Fromm RE Jr, Orr RA, Rotello LC, Horst HM. Guidelines for the inter- and intrahospital transport of critically ill patients. *Crit Care Med* 2004; 32(1): 256-62.

A50   A

A variety of outcomes are possible following either traumatic or non-traumatic brain injury. A vegetative state is characterised by a patient who is 'wakeful without awareness'. Such patients show eye opening and closing mirroring the sleep-wake cycle, have cardiorespiratory stability and exhibit a range of non-purposeful movements, but have no capacity to recognise or interact with the world. This is thought to be explained by severe disruption to the cerebral cortex, but with intact brainstem and thalamic function. The presence of the above features for over 1 month allows the term 'persistent vegetative state' to be used, but this is a diagnostic rather than a prognostic label. The prognosis is influenced by the precipitating event; traumatic causes of brain injury have a better outcome than ischaemic or metabolic causes. The probability of recovery of awareness is less than 1% after 3 months in a non-traumatic vegetative state, and after 12 months in a traumatic vegetative state; the term 'permanent vegetative state' may be used after 12 months, and implies minimal likelihood of improvement [1]. A minimally conscious state is a variant of the persistent vegetative state. Such patients retain some degree of awareness; they may be able to obey a simple command and have limited interaction with their environment (e.g. social smiling, mood disturbance). Coma is a pathological state of eyes-closed unconsciousness from which patients cannot be aroused to wakefulness by stimuli. It is usually temporary (rarely lasting more than a month in the absence of ongoing causes), and may progress to full recovery, death or persistent vegetative state. Brainstem death is characterised by loss of all cranial nerve reflexes, and loss of cardio-respiratory homeostasis. It is assumed that all higher mental function has ceased also; such patients are neither wakeful nor aware. Awareness is preserved in the locked-in syndrome, which may be caused by an insult at the level of the midbrain, such as central pontine myelinosis or basilar artery thrombosis. Quadriplegia and loss of function of the lower cranial nerves may leave the patient almost totally void of means of interaction with the world, despite full awareness. Vertical eye movements and blinking may be preserved.

1. Multi-Society Task Force on PVS. Medical aspects of the persistent vegetative state: parts I and II. *N Engl J Med* 1994; 330: 1499-508, 1572-9.
2. Bernat JL. Chronic disorders of consciousness. *Lancet* 2006; 367: 1181-92.

Paper 2

Type 'K' answers

K51 TFTT

Triamterene is a potassium-sparing diuretic like amiloride and blocks Na^+/K^+ exchange in the distal convoluted tubule. Aminoglycosides and penicillin analogues cause renal potassium wasting. Metolazone is a thiazide diuretic and inhibits Na^+ and Cl^- absorption in the early distal convoluted tubule, meaning more Na^+ is exchanged for K^+ later on in the distal tubule with consequent K^+ loss in the urine.

1. Peck TE, Hill SA, Williams M. *Pharmacology for Anaesthesia and Intensive Care*, 2nd Ed. London: Greenwich Medical Media, 2003.

K52 TTFT

Skin resistance is around 100,000 Ohms when dry, but just 1000 Ohms when wet. If a voltage of 240V is applied, 0.24mA will flow when dry, but 240mA when wet. An AC current of 100mA will cause ventricular fibrillation (VF), but 5A is required to cause sustained asystole. Microshock can be caused by currents as small as 50μA if directly applied to the heart (e.g. saline filled catheter or pacing wire).

1. Soni N. Electrical Injury. *Current Anaesthesia & Critical Care* 2002; 13: 92-6.

K53 TTTT

In general pacing is indicated for symptomatic bradycardia where a documented correlation between the heart rate and the symptoms has been shown and there are no culprit medications which can be stopped. This includes sino-atrial node dysfunction, heart block and carotid sinus dysfunction. In addition, asymptomatic patients with complete heart block merit pacing if ventricular pauses >3s or a heart rate <40bpm are documented. In the setting of acute myocardial infarction, indications for permanent pacing include complete heart block, any symptomatic persistent AV block, and second degree heart block with bundle branch block.

1.   Kaushik V, *et al.* Bradyarrhythmias, temporary and permanent pacing. *Crit Care Med* 2000; 28(10): N121-8.

K54 TFTF

A meta-analysis of studies of outcome of comatose survivors of cardiac arrest has shown that an arrest rhythm of PEA/asystole, anoxic time >5 minutes and CPR time of >25 minutes all predict poor neurological outcome, but with a high rate of false positives (i.e. not suitable as prognostic markers). The absence of pupillary or corneal reflexes, or absent/extensor motor reflexes at 72h post-arrest is invariably predictive of a poor outcome. The predictive value of brain swelling on a CT scan is not known and cannot be relied upon for prognostication.

1.   Wijdicks EFM, *et al.* Practice parameter: prediction of outcome in comatose survivors after cardiopulmonary resuscitation (an evidence-based review). *Neurology* 2006; 67: 203-10.

K55 TFFF

Transthoracic echocardiography is the technique of choice for detecting pericardial fluid, being fast and sensitive in the right hands. A CT scan is likely to be hazardous for this patient and will not alter the need for decompression of the pericardial sac. Intravenous fluid is required to try and maintain right heart filling and cardiac output. Removal of as little as

30ml fluid may give dramatic improvement. Immediate thoracotomy is not mandatory although it may be the management of choice in cardiothoracic centres, and is indicated in the event of deterioration or cardiac arrest.

1. Bersten AD, Soni N. *Oh's Intensive Care Manual,* 5th Ed. Edinburgh: Butterworth-Heinemann, 2003.

K56   FFTF

In major polytrauma it is recognised that coagulopathy, hypothermia and metabolic acidosis are great risks to the patient, and are exacerbated by prolonged surgery. For this reason initial surgery should consist of damage limitation only. This may involve packing a bleeding liver rather than formal resection, debridement of a pancreatic injury rather than pancreaticoduodenectomy, or resecting non-viable bowel and stapling the ends rather than attempting primary re-anastomosis. Re-operation for definitive surgery should take place in the next 24-48 hours if possible, once the patient is warmed, fluid resuscitated and acidosis and coagulopathy have been corrected. Fractures should be stabilised early, since this reduces the rate of ARDS and multiple organ failure. Intramedullary reaming, however, can worsen lung injury and may be best avoided, with external fixation a preferred option. Abdominal closure may provoke abdominal compartment syndrome which has a high mortality. Consideration should be given to leaving the abdomen open as a laparostomy with delayed closure at a later date.

1. Deitch EA, *et al*. Intensive care unit management of the trauma patient. *Crit Care Med* 2006; 34(9): 2294-301.

K57   TTFT

The immediate effects of mannitol may be as a result of reduced haematocrit and improved blood rheology. The high osmolality of the drug also establishes an osmotic gradient between the blood and brain drawing water across areas of intact blood-brain barrier. Mannitol is an osmotic diuretic and can cause volume depletion after an initial increase in intravascular volume which may worsen cardiac failure. The cerebral effect is usually rapid in cases of acutely raised intracranial pressure. Calculated plasma osmolality may not reflect true (measured) osmolality since mannitol is not part of this calculation - it must therefore be measured in the laboratory.

1. Helmy A, Vizcaychipi M, Gupta AK. Traumatic brain injury: intensive care management. *Br J Anaes* 2007; 99 (1): 32-42.

K58   TFFT

Oxygen should be given as soon as available. Hydrocortisone is important in the secondary management but is not time-critical. Epinephrine should be given IM in this dose. Although it may be titrated IV by those experienced in this, this should be done in aliquots of 50-100µg for an adult patient. Leg raising effectively 'autotransfuses' the patient and helps support cardiac output until intravenous access and fluid therapy begins.

1. Working Group of the Resuscitation Council (UK). Emergency treatment of anaphylactic reactions. London: Resuscitation Council (UK), 2008.

K59   FTFF

This history is suggestive of right ventricular infarction. This classically presents as chest pain, hypotension, clear lung fields and distended neck veins. Right atrial pressure is elevated but volume loading may be required to increase right ventricular output. Inotropes such as dobutamine may be required. ST elevation in lead V4R is highly sensitive and specific for RV infarction. Nitrates should be avoided since the right heart is exquisitely sensitive to volume loading and this may precipitate profound hypotension. Thrombolysis is indicated.

1. Horan LG, Flowers MC. Right ventricular infarction: specific requirements of management. *Am Fam Physician* 1999; 60(6): 1727-34.

K60   TFFT

Transfusion-related acute lung injury (TRALI) is caused by the infusion of blood products. Donor antibodies are thought to target host leukocytes causing complement activation, pulmonary leukostasis, capillary leak and acute lung injury. It can be diagnosed if the patient fulfils the standard criteria for acute lung injury and this is temporally related to blood product transfusion. It must be distinguished from anaphylaxis and volume overload. In decreasing order of potential to cause TRALI are: whole blood-derived platelets, fresh frozen plasma (FFP), packed red blood cells, whole blood and apheresis platelet concentrates. Diuretics and corticosteroids are not of benefit.

1.   Silliman C, Ambruso DR, Boshkov LK. Transfusion-related acute lung injury. *Blood* 2005; 105: 2266-73.

K61   FTFT

Intracranial pressure (ICP) measurement is a crude means of estimating cerebral metabolism and blood flow. However, ICP correlates with survival. With severe head injury and ICP <20mmHg, expected mortality is 18%; this rises to 45% >20mmHg, 74% >40mmHg, and 100% >60mmHg [1]. Jugular bulb oxygen saturation ($SjvO_2$) reflects brain tissue oxygen consumption, and one episode of desaturation <50% more than doubles mortality. A fall in $SjvO_2$ may reflect inadequate delivery of oxygen to the brain secondary to systemic causes (hypotension, hypoxia, anaemia, hypocarbia) or cerebral causes (vasospasm, raised ICP). A high mean $SjvO_2$ (>75%) also carries a poor prognosis since dead brain tissue does not extract oxygen. A low arterio-jugular oxygen content difference ($AJDO_2$) suggests poor oxygen extraction by the brain and is associated with a worse outcome [2].

1.   Eker C, *et al.* Improved outcome after severe head injury with a new therapy based on principles for brain volume regulation and preserved microcirculation. *Crit Care Med* 1998; 26(11): 1881-6.
2.   Brain Trauma Foundation; American Association of Neurological Surgeons; Congress of Neurological Surgeons; Joint Section on Neurotrauma and Critical Care, AANS/CNS. Guidelines for the management of severe traumatic brain injury. X. Brain oxygen monitoring and thresholds. *J Neurotrauma* 2007; 24 Suppl 1: S65-70.

K62   FFFF

Recombinant factor VIIa (Novoseven®) is licensed in the United States and UK for the treatment of bleeding in haemophiliacs with antibodies to Factor XIII or IX, and also for patients with acquired Factor VII deficiency. It is also licensed for surgical bleeding prophylaxis in these patient groups. It has been used off-label for many indications including those listed in the question. Although many case reports support its use, there may be an element of publication bias whereby editors are more likely to publish apparently positive results.

1.   Levi M, Peters M, Buller HR. Efficacy and safety of recombinant factor VIIa for treatment of severe bleeding: a systematic review. *Crit Care Med* 2005; 33(4): 883-90.

K63   FFTF

Cardiac output is usually decreased immediately following injury as a result of sympathetic activation increasing systemic and pulmonary vascular resistance. A hypometabolic ('ebb') phase is usual in the first few days following a burn injury (or any major systemic insult), with the hypermetabolic phase supervening around 3 days post-burn. Albumin levels fall, increasing the free fraction of acidic drugs such as benzodiazepines, while α_1-acid glycoprotein levels will be raised, reducing the free fraction of basic drugs such as local anaesthetics and muscle relaxants. Sensitivity to non-depolarising relaxants is reduced from around 1 week post-burn.

1.   Mackie DP. Burns. In: *Oh's Intensive Care Manual*, 5th Ed. Bersten AD, Soni N, Eds. Edinburgh: Butterworth-Heinemann, 2003.

K64   TTTT

The proportion of *Staphylococcus aureus* infections that are methicillin-resistant has risen from 3% to 53% over the last 20 years. Many factors are associated with MRSA infection, including a low nurse to patient ratio, presumably as a result of poorer compliance with barrier nursing procedures. MRSA bacteraemia carries a 14-15% mortality, compared with an 8-9% mortality for methicillin-sensitive strains. Surveillance cultures have been repeatedly demonstrated to lower MRSA infection rates when coupled with appropriate barrier nursing measures. Since most patients are colonised with rather than infected by MRSA, it will not be found unless specifically looked for.

1. Salgado CD, O'Grady N, Farr BM. Prevention and control of antimicrobial-resistant infections in intensive care patients. *Crit Care Med* 2005; 33(10): 2373-82.

K65   TTTT

Left atrial pressure is elevated in mitral stenosis (where a large A-wave will be present), and therefore so is PAOP. In mitral regurgitation the regurgitant V-wave increases mean left atrial pressure also. Massive pulmonary embolism and any cause of increased pulmonary vascular resistance increases the PAOP-left ventricular end-diastolic pressure gradient. If the catheter tip is in West zones I or II, a continuous column of fluid in continuity with the left atrium will not be present throughout the respiratory cycle, since alveolar pressure will exceed pulmonary venous pressure. In this case PAOP will exceed diastolic pulmonary artery pressure, and will overestimate LVEDP.

1. Robin E, *et al.* Clinical relevance of data from the pulmonary artery catheter. *Crit Care* 2006; 10(Suppl 3): S3 (doi:10.1186/cc4830).

K66   FFTT

Passive leg raising has the effect of autotransfusing blood into the central circulation from the venous reservoir of the legs. If elevated to >30°, this should produce an increase in cardiac output after 30s measured by oesophageal Doppler probe if the patient is preload-responsive. Pulmonary artery occlusion pressure has been shown to be a poor predictor of left ventricular end-diastolic volume, and of preload responsiveness. A 'swing on the arterial trace' reflects the greater variation in venous return to the heart caused by transient inspiratory increases in intrathoracic pressure during positive pressure ventilation in patients with an 'empty' circulation. A pulse pressure variation of >13%

has been shown to be a sensitive and specific predictor of increased cardiac output in response to a fluid bolus. A fall in central venous pressure (CVP) of >1mm during spontaneous inspiration has also been shown to predict response to fluid but is difficult to measure in practice. In general, dynamic measures of preload response are superior to traditional static measures such as CVP and PAOP.

1.   Pinsky MR, Payen D. Functional haemodynamic monitoring. *Crit Care* 2005; 9(6): 566-72.

K67   FTTF

A carboxyhaemoglobin level of 10% is insufficient to explain a GCS of 12 and a seizure (smokers may have carboxyhaemoglobin levels of up to 10% with no symptoms). A raised lactate is non-specific, but a normal value excludes significant cyanide toxicity. A serum lactate of >10mmol/L is strongly suggestive of cyanide toxicity in the context of inhalational injury. A central venous blood gas would allow calculation of the arteriovenous oxygen difference, which will be reduced in cyanide toxicity since oxidative phosphorylation and therefore oxygen utilisation at a cellular level is inhibited. Confirmatory evidence of cyanide poisoning may take some time, and treatment should not be delayed if the patient is unwell. Possible antidotes include sodium thiosulphate, hydroxycobalamin and sodium nitrite; sodium nitroprusside is a cause of cyanide toxicity when infused too rapidly.

1.   Baud FJ, Borron SW, Megarbane B, *et al.* Value of lactic acidosis in the assessment of the severity of acute cyanide poisoning. *Crit Care Med* 2002; 30: 2044-50.
2.   Cummings TF. The treatment of cyanide poisoning. *Occup Med (Lond)* 2004; 54(2): 82-5.

K68   TTFT

Benzodiazepines may be administered to ameliorate alcohol withdrawal, although withdrawal symptoms may complicate the prolonged use of these drugs. Patients with cardiopulmonary compromise may suffer from increased oxygen requirements and struggle to clear carbon dioxide generated in part by the stress response; sedatives and analgesics have been shown to reduce both oxygen consumption and autonomic hyperactivity. Provision of sufficient sedation for complete amnesia is mandatory during periods of neuromuscular blockade, although gauging the right level may be difficult. There is increasing evidence that amnesia during critical illness may be associated with a higher incidence of post-traumatic stress disorder, and that preserving awareness during mechanical ventilation may limit this complication. No study has shown amnesia for extended periods to be beneficial in mechanically ventilated intensive care patients.

1. Cullis B, Macnaughton P. Sedation and neuromuscular paralysis in the ICU. *Anaesthesia & Intensive Care Medicine* 2006; 8(1): 32-5.

K69   FFTT

The capnograph trace can be divided into phases I, II, III and IV (see answer to Paper 1, Question A21). Phase III is the plateau phase, which in this case has a steeper slope than normal. In bronchospasm (asthma, COPD), alveolar units with poor ventilation (low V/Q ratio) empty later in expiration than those that are well ventilated. These late-emptying units have a higher CO_2 concentration due to their lower V/Q ratios, and also due to the fact that they empty later in the cardiac cycle and therefore have accrued more CO_2 from the blood. The end-tidal CO_2 is therefore a reflection of those alveoli with the largest time constants (i.e. compliance x resistance). Endobronchial intubation does not cause this waveform; usually the capnograph trace remains normal although the end-tidal CO_2 will steadily rise as alveolar minute volume is greatly reduced.

1. Bhavani-Shankar K, *et al.* Capnometry and anaesthesia. *Can J Anaesth* 1992; 39(6): 617-32.

K70   FFTF

Thrombolysis should be considered for patients with right ventricular compromise and systemic hypotension. The risk of clinically significant bleeding is around 3% with tissue plasminogen activator (TPA). Mortality has not been shown to improve, although right ventricular function has been shown to improve in the first 3 days following thrombolysis. The $S_1Q_3T_3$ pattern on the ECG comprises a prominent S wave in lead I with a Q wave and T wave inversion in lead III. Although this may indicate right ventricular strain it is not in itself an accepted indication for thrombolysis. A hypotensive patient is more seriously ill with a higher mortality risk (24% with right ventricular compromise), and therefore the benefits of thrombolysis may outweigh the risks in this situation, and its use should be considered.

1. Kinane TB, *et al.* Case 7 2008: a 17-year-old girl with chest pain and haemoptysis. *New Engl J Med* 2008; 358: 941-52.

K71 TFTF

Delirium in the ICU has been shown to increase the hazard ratio of death within 6 months by a factor of 3.2. It is experienced by around 80% of mechanically ventilated ICU patients. It is usually recognised in agitated, combative patients, but also occurs in apparently calm patients who may have a hypoactive, withdrawn form of delirium. This latter form is more common, under-recognised and possibly associated with worse outcomes. The CAM-ICU (Confusion Assessment Method for ICU patients) is a delirium assessment tool validated for use in mechanically ventilated ICU patients. Delirium is defined as an acute change or fluctuation in the course of a patient's mental status, plus inattention and either disorganised thinking or an altered level of consciousness. Assessment requires the patient to be sufficiently conscious to respond to a variety of simple questions with a non-verbal signal.

1. Ely EW, *et al.* Evaluation of delirium in critically ill patients: validation of the Confusion Assessment Method for the Intensive Care Unit (CAM-ICU). *Crit Care Med* 2001; 29: 1370-9.
2. Vanderbilt University Medical Center Delirium and Cognitive Impairment Study Group (2008). Delirium and clinical outcomes. Available: http://www.icudelirium.org/delirium/index.html. Last accessed 16 October 2008.

K72 TFFT

The Dopper effect is as stated. An example is the change in observed pitch of sound of a car approaching and passing by a stationary observer. In colour flow Doppler measurement, a red signal indicates flow towards the probe, and a blue signal indicates flow away. Ideally the ultrasound beam should be as near parallel to the direction of blood flow as possible. This is explained by the Doppler equation: $V = C \times \Delta f/2ft \times \cos\theta$, where V = velocity of blood flow, C = speed of sound in soft tissue, Δf = Doppler shift (the difference between received and transmitted [ft] frequency of ultrasound), and θ = angle between direction of blood flow and direction of the ultrasound beam. If θ is 0, $\cos\theta$ is 1, but as θ gets progressively closer to 90° the velocity of blood flow becomes more and more underestimated. At 90° $\cos\theta$ = 0 (velocity is not measured).

1. Donovan KD, Colreavy FB. Echocardiography in intensive care. In: *Oh's Intensive Care Manual*, 5th Ed. Bersten AD, Soni N, Eds. Edinburgh: Butterworth-Heinemann, 2003.

K73 FTFF

Late onset ventilator-associated pneumonia (VAP) can be defined as pneumonia in a mechanically ventilated patient with onset at least 5 days after hospital admission. It is suggested by the presence of new infiltrates on the chest X-ray with other features such as a rising white cell count, pyrexia or hypothermia, increased volume and purulence of tracheobronchial aspirate and worsening indices of oxygenation. Likely pathogens are Gram-negative organisms aspirated from the gastrointestinal tract. After 7 days of mechanical ventilation, the presence of multi-drug resistant organisms is increasingly likely. Unlike early VAP, late VAP increases ICU mortality. While a qualitative sampling process such as blind tracheobronchial aspiration has a high negative predictive value (provided empirical antibiotics have not been started), quantitative methods such as protected specimen brushings are not very specific. Empirical treatment should be with combination therapy for late onset VAP, with coverage of potentially drug-resistant organisms such as *Pseudomonas spp* and *Acinetobacter spp*. Monotherapy with a quinolone would be inadequate in this case.

1. American Thoracic Society; Infectious Diseases Society of America. Guidelines for the management of adults with hospital-acquired, ventilator-associated, and healthcare-associated pneumonia. *Am J Respir Crit Care Med* 2005; 171: 388-416.
2. Ewig S, Bauer T, Torres A. The pulmonary physician in critical care 4: nosocomial pneumonia. *Thorax* 2002; 57: 366-71.

K74   TFTT

Static compliance is calculated as follows: Tidal volume/(Plateau pressure - PEEP). Its calculation therefore requires an end-inspiratory hold to determine plateau pressure. Dynamic compliance is calculated as follows: Tidal volume/(Peak pressure - PEEP), and will be affected by both airway resistance and inspiratory flow rate, as both will alter peak pressure. Since peak pressure is always greater than plateau pressure, it follows that static compliance is always greater than dynamic compliance for a given patient.

1. Jubran A. Monitoring mechanics during mechanical ventilation. *Semin Respir Crit Care Med* 1999; 20(1): 65-79.

K75   TFFT

Tachyarrhythmias in Wolff-Parkinson-White (WPW) syndrome may be either atrioventricular re-entrant tachycardias (AVRTs) or fast atrial fibrillation (AF). AVRTs are caused by a circuit developing between the AV node and the accessory conducting pathway, triggered by an ectopic beat. They can be treated in the same way as atrioventricular non-re-entrant tachycardias (AVNRTs), i.e. vagal manoeuvres, adenosine, verapamil. In fast AF associated with WPW syndrome, however, drugs with AV node-blocking activity such as digoxin, calcium channel blockers and adenosine should be avoided. These drugs reduce conduction through the AV node, meaning that a greater proportion of atrial activity is conducted via the accessory pathway, increasing the ventricular rate and risking ventricular fibrillation. Most cases of fast AF with WPW syndrome are haemodynamically unstable and should receive DC cardioversion. Those which are stable should be treated with drugs that prolong the refractory period of the accessory pathway such as procainamide, sotalol and flecainide. Amiodarone is advocated by many authorities, but has also been blamed for precipitating ventricular fibrillation.

1. Keating L, Morris FP, Brady WJ. Electrocardiographic features of Wolff-Parkinson-White syndrome. *Emerg Med J* 2003; 20: 491-3.

K76   TFFF

This patient is likely to have acute mesenteric ischaemia, a condition which carries a 70% mortality rate. Two thirds of patients are female with a median age of 70 years. The diagnosis should be suspected in patients with a history of cardiovascular disease presenting with severe abdominal pain out of proportion to the physical findings. Arterial embolism, usually from a cardiac source, accounts for 50% of cases, with arterial thrombosis, hypoperfusion states (e.g. shock) and venous thrombosis making up the rest. The most useful laboratory findings are leukocytosis, haemoconcentration and a high anion gap lactic acidosis. Mesenteric angiography is the investigation of choice, but should not delay laparotomy if clinical suspicion is high, since operative delay increases mortality. Abdominal duplex ultrasound and CT are insufficiently sensitive and specific to be of use in the emergency setting. Surgical treatment includes revascularisation and resection of necrotic bowel; thrombolysis is not indicated in this setting. In a less acutely unwell patient, mesenteric angina would be a possibility, and in some cases might be managed conservatively. Such patients typically present with post-prandial abdominal pain which may lead to anorexia and malnutrition. A history of atheromatous disease is usual. Mesenteric angiography in such cases may show areas of stenosis with a well-developed collateral mesenteric circulation.

1. Hirsch AT, *et al.* ACC/AHA 2005 Practice guidelines for the management of patients with peripheral arterial disease. *Circulation* 2006; 113(11): e463-654.

K77   TTTF

Although COPD *per se* (especially emphysema) is associated with increased static compliance of the lungs, in an acute exacerbation hyperinflation is increased due to gas trapping. This means that the patient is breathing at the top of the pressure-volume curve where compliance is greatly reduced. Pulmonary vascular resistance is increased, right heart filling is reduced, and cardiac output falls consequently. Widespread bronchospasm and mucous plugging impose an increased resistive load. As the lungs are hyperinflated, the diaphragm is displaced downwards and is flattened, losing much of its mechanical advantage.

1. Davidson AC. The pulmonary physician in critical care 11: critical care management of respiratory failure resulting from COPD. *Thorax* 2002; 57: 1079-84.

K78   FFFF

The flow-volume loop shown is typical of vocal cord dysfunction (VCD). The inspiratory limb is flattened but the expiratory limb is normal with no 'dip' suggestive of bronchospasm. This diagnosis should be considered in any patient presenting with acute onset shortness of breath. Abnormal adduction of the vocal cords is present during the inspiratory phase but not expiration, causing a variable extrathoracic obstruction. This is commonly mistaken for acute severe asthma, leading to unnecessary intubation and ventilation. In some cases there may be an organic cause such as gastro-oesophageal reflux, but in most this is a functional disorder. It is most common in young adult females and has an association with psychiatric disease. 50% of patients with VCD also have asthma; only a minority of true asthmatics have VCD, however (though many may be misdiagnosed). The diagnosis is confirmed by indirect laryngoscopy which shows complete adduction of the anterior two thirds of the vocal cords during inspiration with a 'glottic chink' posteriorly. Speech therapy and/or psychotherapy are of use in treating the condition. Steroids and bronchodilators are ineffective. Gaseous induction of anaesthesia might be appropriate if suspicion of organic upper airway obstruction is present. The history does not suggest this; there is no history of trauma or foreign body inhalation, and the onset is sudden, excluding infective causes such as acute epiglottitis which becomes symptomatic over a period of hours. In a patient with suspicion of impending upper airway obstruction, awake fibreoptic intubation would be hazardous and risks precipitating complete obstruction (the 'cork in bottle' effect).

1. Borer H, *et al.* Vocal cord dysfunction: an important differential diagnosis of brittle asthma. *Respiration* 2001; 68: 318.

K79 FFFT

A study of DC cardioversion of *de novo* supraventricular tachycardias (mainly fast atrial fibrillation) in ICU surgical patients showed initial restoration of sinus rhythm in just 35% of patients [1]. This was maintained at 48 hours in only 13.5% of patients. Studies in medical (non-ICU) patients have shown much higher success rates (68% in one study [2]). This may be explained by differences in the arrhythmogenic triggering factors at play such as the peri-operative neurohormonal response seen in surgical patients. Successful cardioversion almost always occurs with the first or second shock. In the study quoted no patient was successfully cardioverted who failed to respond to the first three shocks.

1. Mayr A, *et al.* Effectiveness of direct-current cardioversion for treatment of supraventricular tachyarrhythmias, in particular atrial fibrillation, in surgical intensive care patients. *Crit Care Med* 2003; 31(2): 401-5.
2. Arnar DO, Danielsen R. Factors predicting maintenance of sinus rhythm after direct current cardioversion of atrial fibrillation and flutter: a reanalysis with recently acquired data. *Cardiology* 1996; 87(3): 181-8.

K80 TTFT

Numerous trials have confirmed the apparent superiority of percutaneous coronary intervention (PCI) over thrombolysis in the management of ST-elevation myocardial infarction (STEMI), but the overall picture is complex. The advantage of PCI over thrombolysis diminishes rapidly if the 'door-to-balloon time' is >90 minutes, a figure that is achieved readily in clinical trials but less frequently in the real world. Moreover, any mortality benefit from PCI over thrombolysis disappears if the added delay (door-to-balloon time minus door-to-needle time) exceeds 62 minutes. Assuming PCI can be delivered in this time frame it is generally the preferred option, especially if cardiogenic shock is present, the presentation is late (>3h post-symptoms) or the diagnosis of STEMI is in doubt. With late presentations the ability of fibrinolytic drugs to restore vessel patency is greatly reduced, but PCI is much less time-limited in this respect.

1. Boden WE, Eagle K, Granger CB. Reperfusion strategies in acute ST-segment elevation myocardial infarction. *J Am Coll Cardiol* 2007; 50(10): 917-28.

K81 TFTT

Several types of left ventricular assist devices (LVADs) are available. These may be classified as providing pulsatile or non-pulsatile flow, each of which can be further subdivided depending on the mechanism of flow generation. All remove blood from the left atrium or ventricle and pump it into the aorta. Blood flow can be improved by several litres per minute, in contrast to intra-aortic balloon counterpulsation which typically produces only modest increases in cardiac output (although great benefits for the myocardial oxygen supply-demand balance). The LVAD does not oxygenate blood, unlike a cardiac bypass system which takes blood from the right side of the heart and oxygenates it before passing it back to the aorta. While LVADs are typically used as a bridge to transplantation in those with a failing heart, selected patients have been maintained on them for months or years (implantable forms of LVAD exist). Retrospective data suggest that compared with inotrope therapy, LVADs improve renal function and blood pressure in patients awaiting cardiac transplant, and reduce the incidence of post-transplant renal failure and right heart failure [1]. Risks include infection and bleeding secondary to the anticoagulation required to prevent clotting in the extracorporeal circuitry of the LVAD.

1   Bank AJ, *et al*. Effects of left ventricular assist devices on outcomes in patients undergoing heart transplantation. *Ann Thorac Surg* 2000; 69(5): 1369-74.
2. Boehmer JP, Popjes E. Cardiac failure: mechanical support strategies. *Crit Care Med* 2006; 34(9): S268-78.

K82 TFFT

Thrombolysis appears to benefit patients with a recent ischaemic stroke who have had haemorrhage excluded by brain imaging, with lower rates of death and dependency at 3-6 months. This is despite an excess of early and late deaths due to intracerebral haemorrhage. Benefits are maximal if administered within 3 hours of the onset of symptoms, and disappear if therapy is delayed more than 6 hours. In the National Institute of Neurological Disorders and Stroke (NINDS) rt-PA study, the rate of symptomatic intracranial haemorrhage was 6.4% in the treatment group compared with 0.6% for controls [1]. The risk of haemorrhagic transformation is increased if blood pressure is excessively high, and cut-off values of 185mmHg systolic and 110mmHg diastolic have been proposed. Indications for thrombolysis are: ischaemic stroke of clearly defined recent onset; measurable neurological deficit; intracranial haemorrhage excluded by neuroimaging.

1. The National Institute of Neurological Disorders and Stroke Study Group. Tissue plasminogen activator for acute ischaemic stroke. *N Engl J Med* 1995; 333(24): 1581-7.
2. Royal College of Physicians. National clinical guidelines for stroke, 2nd Ed. Prepared by the Intercollegiate Stroke Working Party. London: RCP, 2004.
3. Wardlaw J, del Zoppo G, Yamaguchi T, Berge E. Thrombolysis for acute ischaemic stroke (Cochrane Review). In: *The Cochrane Library*. Chichester, UK: John Wiley and Sons, 2004: Issue 1.

K83   FFTF

The history given of altered sensorium, pyrexia, focal neurological deficit and headache is suggestive of acute encephalitis. The commonest cause of this is *Herpes simplex*, although the differential diagnosis is broad especially in the context of recent foreign travel. Altered sensorium and focal neurological deficit argue against a diagnosis of viral meningitis. A CT brain scan is useful; although it is insensitive for detection of viral encephalitis, it rules out other pathologies such as intracranial haemorrhage or a space-occupying lesion which is necessary prior to lumbar puncture. Magnetic resonance imaging is much more sensitive and may show focal oedema in cases of *Herpes simplex* encephalitis (HSE), especially involving the frontal and temporal lobes. Untreated HSE has a mortality of 70%, mandating immediate intravenous acyclovir on suspicion of the diagnosis. Even with treatment, mortality is 20-30%. Significant neurobehavioral sequalae are common in survivors.

1. Polhill S, Soni M. Encephalitis in the ICU setting. *Current Anaesthesia & Critical Care* 2007; 18: 107-16.

K84   FFFT

In a large, multicentre, multinational observational study of ICU patients meeting predefined criteria for renal replacement therapy, sepsis was the commonest factor associated with acute renal failure (47.5% of patients), while hypovolaemia was associated with 26% of cases. The overall hospital mortality of ICU patients with ARF was 60.3%, compared with a predicted mortality of 45.6%. In this study the overall prevalence of renal failure in ICU patients was 6%, with a variation from 1.4-25.9% depending on the institution. The majority (86%) of survivors were dialysis-independent on discharge from hospital.

1.   Uchino S, Kellum JA, Bellomo R, *et al.* Acute renal failure in critically ill patients: a multinational, multicenter study. *JAMA* 2005; 294(7): 813-8.

K85   FTTT

Stress-related mucosal damage (SRMD) in ICU patients takes the form of an acute erosive gastritis, commonly evident after 24 hours. Important factors in the development of SRMD include compromised gastric mucosal perfusion and acidity of stomach contents. A large prospective study of ICU patients showed an incidence of clinically significant bleeding of 1.5% [1]. ICU mortality is around four times higher in these patients than the general ICU population. Acid suppression with H_2-receptor antagonists has been repeatedly shown to be superior to placebo in preventing this complication of intensive care.

1.   Cook DJ, Fuller HD, Guyatt GH, *et al.* Risk factors for gastrointestinal bleeding in critically ill patients. Canadian Critical Care Trials Group. *N Engl J Med* 1994; 330: 377-81.
2.   Stollman N, Metz DC. Pathophysiology and prophylaxis of stress ulcer in intensive care unit patients. *Journal of Critical Care* 2005; 20: 35-45.

K86 FFFT

'ICU jaundice' is characterised by elevated plasma bilirubin concentration with relatively normal liver enzymes. It commonly presents a week after major surgery or trauma. Ultrasound of the biliary tract should be performed to exclude an obstructive cause. Conventional signs of liver failure such as encephalopathy and asterixis are not present. Histological findings include intrahepatic cholestasis which is thought to be a consequence of uncontrolled production of inflammatory cytokines by Kupffer cells acting on adjacent hepatocytes. No specific treatment is indicated other than of the underlying disease. A raised AST level would raise the possibility of ischaemic hepatitis.

1. Hawker F. Hepatic failure. In: *Oh's Intensive Care Manual.* Bersten AD, Soni N, Eds. Edinburgh: Butterworth-Heinemann, 2003.

K87 FTTF

'Myxoedema coma' is a misnomer, since few patients are comatose. Altered mentation, depression and slowing of thought are common, however. Cool dry skin, non-pitting oedema (myxoedema), hypothermia, constipation and alopecia may all be present. Hyponatraemia is a consequence of reduced free water clearance due to impaired renal blood flow and elevated levels of antidiuretic hormone. Creatine kinase may be elevated as a result of thyroid myopathy, although the exact mechanism is poorly understood. Thyrotrophin (TSH) is usually very high in an attempt to drive thyroid hormone production from an under-performing thyroid gland, except in rare cases of pituitary hypothyroidism.

1. Wall CR. Myxoedema coma: diagnosis and treatment. *Am Fam Phys* 2000; 62: 2485-90.

K88 FFFF

Calculated GFR shows poor agreement with measured GFR in critically ill patients. The Cockroft-Gault formula estimates GFR based on the serum creatinine, height, weight and age of the patient: (140-age) x body weight x 1.73(x0.85 if female)/serum creatinine(mg/dL) x 72 x body surface area. It is validated in patients with chronic renal failure, but tallies less well with measured GFR in critically ill patients. A normal serum creatinine level was shown in one study of critically ill patients to be associated with a measured GFR of <80ml/min in 46% of patients and <60ml/min in 25%. This may be because muscle mass is reduced in this population meaning to such an extent that even with poor renal clearance, creatinine is not elevated above the normal range. GFR can be measured from any timed collection of urine, although a 24-hour collection will average out variations and sampling errors for a more accurate result.

1.   Hoste EA, *et al.* Assessment of renal function in recently admitted critically ill patients with normal serum creatinine. *Nephrol Dial Transplant* 2005; 20: 747-53.

K89   FFTT

The most convincing evidence for a mortality benefit from tight glucose control was provided by a large randomised controlled trial of intensive versus standard insulin therapy in predominantly cardiac surgical ICU patients (in-hospital mortality 10.9% vs. 7.2%) [1]. In this study mortality benefit was seen only in patients requiring ICU care for >5 days. Further analysis showed that the level of glucose control rather than the amount of insulin used conferred the beneficial effects [2]. A similar study in medical ICU patients demonstrated a significant morbidity benefit with tight glycaemic control, but was unable to demonstrate an overall mortality benefit [3]. Mortality was higher in patients staying <3 days, but lower in patients staying >3 days when compared with the control group. Nevertheless, tight glycaemic control was associated with earlier weaning, a lower incidence of renal impairment and faster ICU and hospital discharge. One caveat of these trials is that very tight glucose control was used in the treatment arms (4.6-6.1mmol/L [80-110mg/dL]). There is an appreciable risk of hypoglycaemia with such tight control especially if enteral feeding is interrupted. Even in these studies the incidence of hypoglycaemia was much higher in the treatment groups, and it can be assumed that outside the rigorous protocol of a clinical trial monitoring may be less stringent and hypoglycaemia more common. Most episodes of hypoglycaemia were related to the unplanned interruption of enteral feeding [2].

1. van den Berghe G, *et al*. Intensive insulin therapy in the critically ill patients. *N Engl J Med* 2001; 345(19): 1359-67.

2. van den Berghe G, *et al*. Outcome benefit of intensive insulin therapy in the critically ill: Insulin dose versus glycemic control. *Crit Care Med* 2003; 31(2): 359-66.

3. van den Berghe G, Wilmer A, Hermans G, *et al*. Intensive insulin therapy in the medical ICU. *N Engl J Med* 2006; 354: 449-61.

K90   TFTF

The Surviving Sepsis Campaign (SSC) is a consensus endeavour by members of 11 international organisations with expertise in the management of sepsis. A series of (recently updated) evidence-based guidelines have been produced by the organisation with the aim of reducing mortality from sepsis [1]. The main points from this guideline have been distilled into two 'sepsis care bundles' to be implemented within 6 and 24 hours of the recognition of a septic patient. The 6-hour bundle is a package of resuscitation measures. Early (within 1 hour) administration of antibiotics after blood culture, aggressive fluid therapy guided by serum lactate, central venous pressure and central or mixed venous oxygen saturation, and appropriate use of vasopressors are the key aims. Activated protein C administration is part of the 24-hour bundle for patients satisfying the criteria.

1. Dellinger RP, *et al* for the International Surviving Sepsis Campaign Guidelines Committee. Surviving Sepsis Campaign: International guidelines for management of severe sepsis and septic shock: 2008. *Crit Care Med* 2008; 36(1): 296-327.

K91   TFTF

Standardised definitions of the systemic inflammatory response syndrome (SIRS), sepsis, severe sepsis and septic shock were proposed by the American College of Chest Physicians/Society of Critical Care Medicine consensus conference in 1992 [1], and updated more recently [2]. SIRS requires two of the following: heart rate >90bpm; white cell count >12,000/mm^3 or <4000/mm^3 or >10% bands (immature neutrophils) on the blood film; respiratory rate >20 breaths/min or $PaCO_2$ <4.3kPa (32.7mmHg); temperature >38°C or <36°C. Sepsis is the presence of SIRS in the context of infection. A positive blood culture is not required, although clinical evidence of infection must exist. In this case the history and radiological evidence are sufficient. Severe sepsis is the presence of sepsis with hypotension, hypoperfusion or organ dysfunction. In this case the raised lactate and base deficit are indicators of hypoperfusion. Septic shock is defined as sepsis-induced hypotension persisting despite adequate fluid resuscitation. This patient has just arrived in the Emergency Room and has not yet been fluid resuscitated.

1.   Bone RC, *et al*. Definitions for sepsis and organ failure and guidelines for the use of innovative therapies in sepsis. The ACCP/SCCM Consensus Conference Committee. American College of Chest Physicians/Society of Critical Care Medicine. *Chest* 1992; 101(6): 1644-55.

2.   Levy MM, *et al*. 2001 SCCM/ESICM/ACCP/ATS/SIS International Sepsis Definitions Conference. *Intensive Care Med* 2003; 29: 530-38.

K92   TTFT

HFOV involves the delivery of high frequency breaths (around 5Hz) of low tidal volume (typically 1-3ml/kg, although this value cannot be directly set). Set values are the frequency, I:E ratio, driving pressure and mean airway pressure. Peak airway pressure is reduced compared with conventional ventilation, but end-expiratory lung volume is higher and mean airway pressure is usually higher. An early increased improvement in oxygenation is typical but this is often not sustained beyond the first 24 hours. In a randomised controlled trial of HFOV in surgical patients [1] meeting the criteria for ARDS, no significant difference in mortality was demonstrated (although the study was not powered for this purpose). Arterial CO_2 tends to run higher in patients ventilated with HFOV, but not to a clinically important degree.

1. Kao KC, *et al.* High frequency oscillatory ventilation for surgical patients with acute respiratory distress syndrome. *J Trauma* 2006; 61: 837-43.
2. Derdak S, *et al.* High-frequency oscillatory ventilation for acute respiratory distress syndrome in adults: a randomized, controlled trial. *Am J Respir Crit Care Med* 2002; 166: 801-8.

K93   FTFT

Hypoxia is an early finding present in over 90% of patients with an amniotic fluid embolism. This may be due to V/Q mismatching, cardiogenic pulmonary oedema secondary to left ventricular dysfunction or bronchospasm; the latter occurs in only 15% of cases. Hypotension is a universal finding. Shock in the early stages is most likely to be due to cardiogenic and obstructive causes, while later a distributive 'septic' picture supervenes. Disseminated intravascular coagulation occurs in 83% of patients. Half of these become coagulopathic within 4 hours of the onset of cardiopulmonary symptoms. 85% of survivors have some form of residual neurological deficit including seizures and altered mentation.

1. Moore J, Baldisseri MR. Amniotic fluid embolism. *Crit Care Med* 2005; 33(10): S279-85.

K94   FTFF

Non-steroidal anti-inflammatory drugs (NSAIDs) inhibit cyclo-oxygenase reducing the formation of thromboxane A_2, prostacyclin (PGI_2) and prostaglandins PGE_2, $PGF_{2\alpha}$ and PGD_2 from arachidonic acid. In susceptible individuals (a small proportion of asthmatics), clinically significant bronchospasm may occur as more arachidonic acid is diverted to leukotriene production. NSAIDs are highly protein bound and may displace warfarin from its albumin binding site. They have a small volume of distribution. NSAIDs are metabolised by the liver either by hydrolysis of conjugation, and the (mainly inactive) metabolites are renally excreted.

1. Analgesics. In: *Pharmacology for Anaesthesia and Intensive Care*, 2nd Ed. Peck TE, Hill SA, Williams M. London: Greenwich Medical Media, 2003.

K95   FFTT

Corneal microdeposits are the commonest complication of treatment, occurring in over 90% of patients. Pulmonary toxicity may occur acutely in the intensive care patient treated with amiodarone. This may be due to immunologically-mediated hypersensitivity, and appears to be more common in patients with pre-existing lung disease and in those undergoing cardiac surgery. Acute respiratory distress syndrome may be precipitated or exacerbated, and bronchiolitis obliterans organising pneumonia (BOOP) may develop. Mild elevation of hepatic transaminases occurs in around 25% of patients; acute hepatotoxocity is a rare but recognised complication of intravenous amiodarone loading. Neurological side effects include tremor, ataxia and peripheral neuropathy. These are related to the dose and duration of therapy.

1. Vassallo P, Trohman RG. Prescribing amiodarone: an evidence-based review of clinical indications. *JAMA* 2007; 298(11): 1312-22.
2. Ashrafian H, Davey P. Is amiodarone an underrecognized cause of acute respiratory failure in the ICU? *Chest* 2001; 120: 275-82.

K96   TFFT

In the equation given, C = drug concentration in the plasma, C_0 = initial concentration, e = natural log, k = the elimination rate constant and t = time. This is an example of first order kinetics where the drug is eliminated from the plasma at a rate proportional to its concentration. This contrasts with zero order metabolism, where the rate of elimination would be independent of concentration (a straight line). A one compartment model is shown, with the drug being theoretically eliminated directly from the plasma (the central compartment). In reality, most drugs are best described by a two- or three-compartment model, where an initial steep decline (redistribution among vessel-rich tissues) is followed by a more gradual decline (redistribution to less well-perfused tissues/elimination from the body). This is best represented graphically as a semi-logarithmic plot with $\log_{10}$concentration on the Y axis. The difference between points A and B is the half-life ($t_{1/2}$), the time taken for the plasma concentration of the drug to fall by 50%. The time constant (T) is the time it would take for the concentration of the drug in the plasma to reach zero if elimination continued at the initial rate. It is related to the half-life by the formula $t_{1/2} = 0.693T$. K is the elimination rate constant, which is the reciprocal of the time constant.

1. Smith TC. Pharmacokinetics. In: *Fundamentals of Anaesthesia*, 2nd Ed. Pinnock C, Lin T, Smith T, Eds. London: Greenwich Medical Media, 2003.

K97   TFTT

Cardiac output measurement using lithium dilution requires delivery of a bolus of lithium chloride through a central or peripheral line which is measured through arterial sampling. It is unsuitable for patients taking maintenance lithium since this alters the background concentration in the plasma and causes an overestimation of cardiac output. Drift of the measurement electrode occurs in the presence of atracurium; a previous bolus dose is not a contraindication to use, however, as long as it is not in circulation at the time of measurement. Since lithium distributes in the plasma, measurement of its concentration will be affected by the packed cell volume, and a correction based on the haemoglobin concentration is required to compensate for this.

1. Jonas M, Hett D, Morgan J. Real time, continuous monitoring of cardiac output and oxygen delivery. *Int J Intensive Care* 2002; 9(1): 33-42.

K98   TFTF

In continuous venovenous haemofiltration (CVVH), ultrafiltration occurs across a porous membrane. Increasing the rate of blood flow through the circuit increases the transmembrane pressure across the filter and therefore increases ultrafiltrate production and resultant solute clearance by convection. Pre-dilution involves addition of replacement fluid into the circuit before passage through the filter. Since the addition of this fluid dilutes the concentration of molecules requiring clearance (such as urea), clearance is less efficient per unit volume of ultrafiltrate. However, this is offset by the fact that: i) increased pump speeds can be achieved due to reduced viscosity, and ii) the filtration fraction can be increased as plasma oncotic pressure (which opposes hydrostatic filtration pressure) is reduced by the dilution. Increasing the surface area of the filter increases ultrafiltration and improves clearance of solutes, but means a greater volume of blood circulating outside the body at any given time. Arteriovenous haemofiltration is no more efficient than venovenous haemofiltration.

1.   Clarke WR, Ronco C. CRRT efficiency and efficacy in relation to solute size. *Kidney International* 1999; 56: S3-7.
2.   Hall NA, Fox AJ. Renal replacement therapies in critical care. *Continuing Education in Anaesthesia, Critical Care & Pain* 2006; 6: 197-202.

K99   TTTT

In a large multi-centre snapshot study of all adverse incidents reported in 205 ICUs worldwide, over a 24-hour period [1], the overall incident rate was 38.8 events per 100 patient days. The commonest adverse event related to displacement of catheters, lines and drains. Factors associated with increased incidence of adverse events included severity of illness, level of care required, Sequential Organ Failure Assessment (SOFA) score and length of stay on the ICU. Patients receiving renal replacement therapy and mechanical ventilation were also at increased risk of adverse events. Interestingly, the patient-to-nurse ratio was not shown to be a significant factor in this study.

1.   Valentin A, *et al*. Patient safety in intensive care: results from the multinational Sentinel Events Evaluation (SEE) study. *Int Care Med* 2006; 32: 1591-8.

K100   FFFT

Persistent vegetative state is essentially wakefulness without awareness. Patients must be shown to lack awareness of themselves and their environment; they are considered unable to think, perceive, or feel emotions. They may display a wide range of spontaneous movements including eye opening and closing following patterns of sleep and wakefulness, roving eye movements and nystagmus, non-purposeful limb movements and vocalisation, as well as flexion withdrawal from noxious stimuli. Cardiorespiratory function is usually well preserved. Evidence of sustained purposeful movements, interaction with others, or language comprehension rule out the diagnosis. Persistent vegetative state implies a clinical state that has been present for at least 4 weeks; a permanent vegetative state implies a prediction that things will not improve.

1. Royal College of Physicians. The vegetative state: guidance on diagnosis and management. London: Royal College of Physicians, 2003.

Paper 3

Type 'A' questions

A1 A 51-year-old man presents with abdominal pain. A CT of the abdomen shows severe necrotising pancreatitis. Routine bloods show a calcium of 4.5mmol/l (18mg/dL). He is lethargic and confused. Which one of the following is FALSE?

a. Rapid intravenous fluids are indicated.
b. Frusemide is a useful treatment for hypercalcaemia.
c. Emergency parathyroidectomy may be required.
d. Steroids effectively treat hypercalcaemia where malignancy is the underlying cause.
e. A parathyroid adenoma is the most likely cause of this man's hypercalcaemia.

A2 A 28-year-old obstetric patient is receiving treatment for severe pre-eclampsia. She is referred to the ICU 1 day post partum with decreased consciousness. On examination she has a GCS of 13 and is confused and listless, with grade 4 power in all four limbs. She is flushed, bradycardic and nauseous. Her ECG shows prolongation of the PR and QT intervals. The 'best-fit' diagnosis is:

a. Intracerebral haemorrhage.
b. Peripartum sepsis.
c. Local anaesthetic toxicity.
d. Hypermagnesaemia.
e. None of the above.

A3 The following are consequences of therapeutic (32-34°C) hypothermia EXCEPT:

a. A 7% fall in cerebral metabolic rate for each 1°C fall in temperature.
b. Decreased reabsorption of solutes by the kidney.
c. Hypoglycaemia.
d. Increased incidence of ventilator-associated pneumonia.
e. Prolonged prothrombin time.

A4 A 19-year-old man is ejected through the front window of a car during a high speed impact and is brought into hospital by the paramedics. The primary survey should include the following points EXCEPT:

a. Use of airway adjuncts if indicated.
b. Control of external haemorrhage.
c. Cervical spine assessment.
d. Pupillary light reflex determination.
e. Percussion of the chest.

A5 Regarding penetrating abdominal injury the following are true EXCEPT:

a. The most common cause of death in the first 24h is haemorrhage.
b. Peritonitis in a haemodynamically stable patient is an indication for laparotomy.
c. The most commonly injured organ in penetrating stab wounds is the liver.
d. Chest X-ray is an insensitive test for diaphragmatic injury.
e. A negative FAST scan has a high negative predictive value for injury requiring laparotomy.

A6 Which of the following is NOT a feature of the abdominal compartment syndrome?

a. Increased pulmonary vascular resistance.
b. Reduced cardiac output.
c. Oliguria.
d. Raised intracranial pressure.
e. Reduced pulmonary artery occlusion pressure.

A7 A 33-year-old woman is admitted to the ICU with pneumonia on a background of varying neurological symptoms with a relapsing and remitting course. She is noted to have weakness and tingling in her legs, and has dysarthria and occulomotor signs. She complains of being tired all the time. Analysis of cerebrospinal fluid shows protein 0.7g/L, glucose 4.5mmol/L [81.8mg/dL] (plasma glucose 5.1mmol/L [92.7mg/dL]) and oligoclonal bands. The MOST LIKELY diagnosis is:

a. Myasthenia gravis.
b. Viral meningitis.
c. Guillain-Barré syndrome.
d. Aseptic meningitis.
e. Multiple sclerosis.

A8 In the management of status epilepticus in adults the following are true EXCEPT:

a. Buccal midazolam 10mg is an alternative to rectal diazepam.
b. Phenytoin should be given in a dose of 15-18mg/kg as a rapid IV bolus.
c. Lorazepam is preferred to diazepam if intravenous access is present.
d. Ideally serum levels should be measured to guide thiopentone infusion.
e. 'Thiopentone coma' should be titrated to burst suppression on the EEG.

A9 The following are common laboratory features of toxic megacolon EXCEPT:

a. Metabolic alkalosis.
b. Hypokalaemia.
c. Raised haematocrit.
d. Anaemia.
e. Leukocytosis with left shift.

A10 A 37-year-old man is transferred to the ICU following a motorbike accident. A CT thorax scan an hour earlier showed three fractured ribs on the left side of the chest, severe pulmonary contusions, and a pelvic fracture (awaiting fixation). Shortly after arrival on ICU, he develops severe respiratory distress over a few minutes. His BP falls to 80/50mm Hg, and he develops a tachycardia (HR 140bpm). Your first priority would be:

a. Immediate intubation and ventilation.
b. Rapid infusion of 1L crystalloid and assess response.
c. Urgent evaluation of the chest for signs of tension pneumothorax.
d. Arrange an urgent surgical opinion.
e. Noradrenaline infusion.

A11 Regarding the usefulness of intracranial pressure (ICP) monitoring in patients with traumatic brain injury which ONE of the following is TRUE?

a. Outcome is improved in patients who respond to ICP-lowering therapies.
b. If the CT scan is normal ICP monitoring is not required.
c. ICP-lowering therapies can safely be given empirically (without ICP monitoring).
d. Cerebral perfusion pressure can be monitored without ICP measurement.
e. Haematoma requiring surgical evacuation occurs as a consequence of ICP monitoring in <0.01% of patients.

A12 Regarding unstable fractures of the pelvis which ONE of the following options is TRUE?

a. Falls from a great height are the commonest cause of injury.
b. Mortality is as high as 45% in haemodynamically unstable patients.
c. Associated intra-abdominal injury is unusual.
d. Pulmonary embolism from pelvic deep vein thrombosis is the commonest cause of death.
e. Arterial embolisation has no role in the management of pelvic bleeding.

A13 Which is the TRUE statement regarding the anaesthetic management of a patient with major burns?

a. Awake fibreoptic intubation is the technique of choice in the patient with stridor following inhalational injury.
b. A high ventilator minute volume will be required.
c. Intramuscular morphine is ideal supplemental analgesia for burns dressing changes.
d. Non-depolarising muscle relaxants should be given in small doses.
e. Theatre temperature should be maintained at 37°C.

A14 A 78-year-old lady is found on the floor at home and is brought to hospital. An initial CT brain scan is normal and a presumptive diagnosis of ischaemic stroke is made with secondary hypothermia. She is admitted to the ICU for mechanical ventilation in view of her reduced GCS. Thyroid function tests include: TSH 25mU/L (normal 0.5-6mU/L), free T4 2pmol/L (normal 10-26pmol/L), T3 0.7nmol/L (normal 1.2-3nmol/L). The most likely diagnosis is:

a. Pituitary apoplexy.
b. Sick euthyroid syndrome.
c. Primary hypothyroidism.
d. Overdose of amiodarone.
e. Viral thyroiditis.

A15 Assuming that VO_2 can be accurately determined, which of the following pieces of additional information is NOT required to calculate cardiac output using the Fick principle?

a. PaO_2.
b.   Mixed venous oxygen saturation.
c. SaO_2.
d. VCO_2.
e.   Haemoglobin concentration.

A16 A 42-year-old woman is admitted to the ICU generally unwell 1 week following abdominal surgery. She is oliguric, hypotensive (BP 80/35mmHg) and tachycardic (HR 130bpm). An oesophageal Doppler probe is sited, showing: flow time (corrected) 380ms, peak velocity 110cm/s, stroke volume 90ml. Which of the following statements is TRUE?

a.   A fluid challenge should be administered.
b.   Cardiac contractility is impaired.
c.   A cautious dose of frusemide should be given.
d.   The measured (uncorrected) flow time will be greater than 380ms.
e.   The data are consistent with massive pulmonary embolism.

A17 Regarding electrical temperature measurement which ONE of the following statements is FALSE?

a.   A thermistor measures temperature using the Seebeck effect.
b.   The resistance of a platinum thermometer increases linearly with increasing temperature.
c.   A thermocouple can measure temperatures up to 1600°C.
d.   A radiation thermometer utilises Planck's law.
e.   A thermistor is a type of semiconductor.

A18 A 78-year-old man is ventilated on the ICU with diffuse brain injury following a fall. He has significant renal impairment (baseline creatinine clearance 22ml/min), as well as sick sinus syndrome for which he is awaiting implantation of a permanent pacemaker. He has a proven allergy to egg protein. Which of the following sedative agents would be most suitable in this case?

a. Midazolam.
b. Propofol.
c. Etomidate.
d. Clonidine.
e. Ketamine.

A19 Regarding the 12-lead ECG the following are true EXCEPT:

a. The scale on the vertical axis is 0.1mV/mm.
b. The QT interval is the time from the start of the QRS complex to the end of the T wave.
c. A cardiac monitor has a broader frequency range than an ECG machine.
d. Lead I measures the potential difference between the left and right arms.
e. The amplitude of the measured ECG signal is much smaller than the actual biological potential across the heart.

A20 A 28-year-old fit and well nurse requiring elective femoral hernia repair is anaesthetised with propofol, atracurium and sevoflurane and her trachea is intubated. Thirty minutes into the procedure she becomes progressively more difficult to ventilate. Her BP falls to 60/40mmHg, her HR is 150bpm and widespread bronchospasm is heard on auscultation of the chest. The MOST LIKELY diagnosis is:

a. Anaphylaxis to atracurium.
b. Vagal reaction to surgical stimulation.
c. Laryngospasm.
d. Latex allergy.
e. Pneumothorax.

A21 A 68-year-old man is admitted to the ICU with septic shock. A few days later he is clinically improving but becomes increasingly agitated and hyper-aroused. A diagnosis of ICU delirium is made. The most appropriate pharmacological intervention would be:

a. Low-dose propofol infusion titrated to the level of arousal.
b. Night sedation with trazodone.
c. Intravenous haloperidol 0.5-10mg.
d. Intravenous lorazepam 0.05-0.1mg/kg.
e. Maintenance of a normal sleep-wake cycle.

A22 Which statement regarding Lundberg waves is FALSE?

a. Three Lundberg waves are described.
b. Type A waves have a duration of 5-20 seconds.
c. Type B waves have the shortest duration.
d. Type C waves have the lowest amplitude.
e. Type A waves are never benign.

A23 An 81-year-old man develops sudden shortness of breath on the orthopaedic ward 1 week after a right total knee replacement. A history of previous deep vein thrombosis following left total knee replacement 2 years ago is noted. On examination he is tachycardic (110bpm) and tachypnoeic (23 breaths per minute). Blood tests reveal an arterial PaO_2 of 6.5kPa (49mmHg) and a $PaCO_2$ of 4.4kPa (33mmHg) on room air. D-dimer is <250ng/ml, and troponin T is 0.5ng/ml (normal range <0.1ng/ml). An ECG shows right axis deviation. Which statement is TRUE?

a. The pretest probability of pulmonary embolism is low.
b. The normal D-dimer excludes a diagnosis of pulmonary embolism.
c. A V/Q scan is a useful investigation in this case.
d. CT contrast arteriography has low specificity for the detection of pulmonary embolism.
e. The elevated troponin is against the diagnosis of pulmonary embolism.

A24 One hour following rapid sequence induction of anaesthesia for appendicectomy a 15-year-old boy is becoming increasingly unwell. On examination, he has a temperature of 39.8°C and a sinus tachycardia (HR 135bpm). Arterial blood gas analysis reveals hyperkalaemia and a metabolic acidosis. The most appropriate treatment is:

a. Intravenous analgesia.
b. Intravenous antibiotics.
c. Paracetamol for its antipyretic action.
d. Propofol bolus to deepen anaesthesia.
e. Intravenous dantrolene.

A25 Which ONE of the following will increase plateau pressure in a patient receiving continuous mandatory ventilation (CMV) for community-acquired pneumonia?

a. Increasing the I:E ratio to 2:1.
b. A decelerating flow pattern.
c. An accelerating flow pattern.
d. Increasing the inspiratory flow rate.
e. Increasing the set tidal volume.

A26 The following drugs are known to cause thrombocytopaenia with the exception of:

a. Heparin.
b. Linezolid.
c. Vancomycin.
d. Sulphonamides.
e. Fentanyl.

A27 A 44-year-old woman with acute severe asthma requires intubation and ventilation following failure of maximal medical treatment. At the time of intubation she has the following observations: BP of 150/90mmHg, HR of 110bpm, RR of 28 breaths per minute. Following intubation she is sedated with a propofol infusion running at 150mg/h and alfentanil at 2mg/h. Over the next 30 minutes a steady cardiovascular deterioration occurs with a fall in BP to 85/65mmHg, and a rise in HR to 130bpm (sinus tachycardia). Clinical examination is unremarkable other than the presence of diffuse expiratory wheeze in both lung fields. The most appropriate action to restore cardiovascular stability is:

a.   Reduce the rate of the propofol infusion.
b.   Commence a noradrenaline infusion.
c.   Stop the aminophylline infusion.
d.   Disconnect the ventilator.
e.   Insert a large-bore cannula in the second intercostal space in the mid-clavicular line.

A28 A 27-year-old brittle asthmatic develops wheeze and dyspnoea during labour. She also has a small post-partum haemorrhage requiring pharmacological control. The following drugs may be safely used EXCEPT:

a.   Prednisolone.
b.   Syntocinon.
c.   Methylxanthines.
d.   Prostaglandin F2a.
e.   Nebulised ß2 agonists.

A29 The following physiological changes occur in the proned patient with acute respiratory distress syndrome (ARDS) EXCEPT:

a. Perfusion is largely redistributed to the ventral lung.
b. Ventilation is more homogenously distributed.
c. A reduction in physiological shunt occurs.
d. Compression of dorsal lung regions by the heart is reduced.
e. Anterior chest wall compliance is decreased.

A30 A 28-year-old previously well woman is seen in the Emergency Room with sudden onset palpitations. The ECG shows atrial fibrillation with a ventricular rate of 140bpm. On examination she complains of a feeling of breathlessness but is able to talk in sentences. Her BP is 100/70mmHg, SpO_2 is 99% on 6L/min oxygen. The most appropriate first-line treatment of her arrhythmia would be:

a. Oral digoxin 250-500µg over 30 minutes.
b. Intravenous metoprolol 2.5-5mg over 1 minute.
c. Intravenous flecainide 100-150mg over 30 minutes.
d. Synchronised DC shock under sedation or anaesthesia.
e. Intravenous verapamil 5mg intravenous bolus.

A31 Which of the following best distinguishes non-ST-segment-elevation myocardial infarction (NSTEMI) from unstable angina?

a. Severe chest pain.
b. ST depression in two or more contiguous leads on the ECG.
c. Raised troponin level.
d. Chest pain lasting more than 15 minutes.
e. Previous confirmed myocardial infarction.

A32 A 65-year-old man is ventilated on the ICU after an emergency laparotomy for a perforated sigmoid diverticulum. He has critical aortic stenosis and is being considered for an aortic valve replacement. Which of the following is NOT an appropriate management strategy?

a. Maintenance of a high left ventricular preload.
b. Swift cardioversion of any atrial fibrillation that develops.
c. Intra-aortic balloon counterpulsation.
d. Use of vasopressors to elevate systemic vascular resistance.
e. Avoidance of all diuretics.

A33 A 27-year-old woman presents to the Emergency Room 1 month after giving birth. She complains of a severe headache which has been getting steadily worse over the last 3 weeks. Previous medical history is unremarkable except for a previous miscarriage. On examination she is drowsy (GCS 14), but has no focal neurological deficit. Papilloedema is visible on fundoscopy. The headache is not relieved by changes in posture. A CT brain scan shows no abnormality. Cerebrospinal fluid analysis is also normal. The most likely diagnosis is:

a. Post-dural puncture headache.
b. Tension headache.
c. Cerebral venous sinus thrombosis.
d. Subarachnoid haemorrhage.
e. Normal pressure hydrocephalus.

A34 A 45-year-old man has been ventilated on the ICU for 2 weeks for a community-acquired pneumonia. He is proving difficult to wean despite adequate nutrition, good gas exchange and correction of his electrolytes. He appears to have developed weakness of his arms and legs, and a diagnosis of critical illness polyneuromyopathy is entertained. Which of the following features is NOT consistent with this diagnosis?

a. Ventilation for >7 days.
b. Flaccid quadriparesis.
c. Elevated serum creatinine kinase.
d. Extensor plantars and hyperreflexia.
e. Four twitches of equal height with train-of-four nerve stimulation.

A35 Which one of the following requires antimicrobial treatment in a catheterised ICU patient in the absence of other clinical indicators?

a. Candida isolated from urine culture.
b. Pyuria.
c. Urine culture showing >10^3 colony forming units/ml bacteria.
d. Positive urine dipstick for leukocyte esterase and/or nitrate.
e. None of the above.

A36 A 33-year-old woman presents with right upper quadrant pain and generalised abdominal swelling. She is previously well and takes no medication other than oral contraception. Past medical history is unremarkable apart from a deep vein thrombosis in pregnancy. Hepatomegaly, ascites and peripheral oedema are present on clinical examination. Ascitic fluid analysis reveals a neutrophil count of 10/mm^3 and a serum-to-ascites albumin gradient of 1.3. 24-hour urine protein concentration is 90mg/L. She denies alcohol excess. The most likely diagnosis from the list below is:

a. Acute alcoholic hepatitis.
b. Budd-Chiari syndrome.
c. Spontaneous bacterial peritonitis.
d. Metastatic disease.
e. Nephrotic syndrome.

A37 A 65-year-old man is admitted to the ICU following emergency abdominal aortic aneurysm repair. Past medical history includes ischaemic heart disease, congestive cardiac failure and benign prostatic hypertrophy. On day 3 liver function tests show an aspartate aminotransferase level of 3,400U/L, a lactate dehydrogenase level of 5,500IU/L and a bilirubin of 52µmol/L (3.04mg/dL). Ultrasound of the biliary tract is unremarkable. The most likely diagnosis is:

a. ICU jaundice.
b. Acalculous cholecystitis.
c. Intravascular haemolysis.
d. Ischaemic hepatitis.
e. Transfusion reaction.

A38 The following drugs require dose modification in renal failure (creatinine clearance <20ml/min) EXCEPT:

a. Tazocin® (tazobactam + piperacillin).
b. Digoxin.
c. Atenolol.
d. Amiodarone.
e. Metformin.

A39 Which of the following is both a sensitive and specific marker of nutritional status in the critically ill patient?

a. Serum albumin.
b. Triceps skin fold thickness.
c. Serial measurement of body mass.
d. Creatinine height index.
e. None of the above.

A40 A 22-year-old man is admitted to the ICU with cocaine toxicity. He is agitated with a HR of 130bpm (sinus tachycardia on the ECG) and a BP of 200/120mmHg. The LEAST appropriate therapy would be:

a. Labetalol.
b. Lorazepam.
c. Phentolamine.
d. Atenolol.
e. Midazolam.

A41 A 26-year-old man is brought to the Emergency Room following a night out. His friends say he has "taken something" in a nightclub and was previously "high". Now he has a GCS of 5. On examination he is a muscular young man, BP is 90/45mmHg and HR is 40bpm. The ECG shows a sinus bradycardia. His temperature is 34.5°C. Arterial blood gas analysis shows a mild respiratory acidosis. There is no response to intravenous naloxone. The emergency physician decides to intubate the patient without sedation, but on direct laryngoscopy he becomes violently agitated. The most likely drug ingested is:

a. 3,4-methylene-dioxymethamphetamine ('ecstasy').
b. Phencyclidine.
c. Ketamine.
d. Gamma-hydroxybutyrate.
e. Heroin.

A42 The following parameters are directly set by the operator of a high frequency oscillatory ventilator EXCEPT:

a. Frequency.
b. Tidal volume.
c. I:E ratio.
d. Driving pressure.
e. Mean airway pressure.

A43 The following are true of the syndrome of haemolysis, elevated liver enzymes and low platelets (HELLP) in pregnancy EXCEPT:

a. Schistocytes are seen on the blood film.
b. Lactate dehydrogenase is elevated.
c. By definition HELLP syndrome occurs in association with pre-eclampsia.
d. Delivery of the foetus is the mainstay of treatment.
e. Hypoglycaemia and acute liver failure are uncommon.

A44 A patient on the ICU is on low-dose aspirin following a myocardial infarction 2 years previously. Which one of the following statements is FALSE?

a. Aspirin has greater effect on platelet cyclo-oxygenase than endothelial cyclo-oxygenase in low doses.
b. In high doses (>600mg) aspirin is a more effective analgesic than most other non-steroidal anti-inflammatory drugs (NSAIDs).
c. Aspirin irreversibly inhibits platelet cyclo-oxygenase.
d. Aspirin may potentiate the effect of warfarin.
e. Haemodialysis is a useful treatment for overdose.

A45 Regarding the hepatic clearance of drugs all the following are true EXCEPT:

a. Drugs with a high extraction ratio exhibit flow-dependent metabolism.
b. Midazolam has a low extraction ratio.
c. Enzyme induction significantly increases clearance of drugs with a low extraction ratio.
d. Phenytoin has a low extraction ratio.
e. A drug with a high extraction ratio will have low bioavailability.

A46 A 44-year-old patient with sickle cell disease is transferred to the ICU for observation following a laparotomy. He is prone to sickling crises. Appropriate management of this patient should include all of the following measures EXCEPT:

a. Good hydration.
b. Exchange transfusion to maintain HbS levels of <15%.
c. Maintenance of normothermia.
d. Avoidance of hypoxaemia.
e. Chest physiotherapy.

A47 A 55-year-old man on the ICU develops *Clostridium difficile* diarrhoea following a course of ciprofloxacin for community-acquired pneumonia. He is initially treated with enteral metronidazole but has large nasogastric aspirates and is thought to have an ileus. The most appropriate treatment for his infection is:

a. Oral vancomycin.
b. Intravenous metronidazole.
c. Intravenous vancomycin.
d. Probiotics.
e. Intravenous immunoglobulin.

A48 A 72-year-old man with chronic renal impairment is admitted to the ICU following an emergency laparotomy. During his stay he develops fast atrial fibrillation and is placed on maintenance amiodarone therapy. He subsequently develops systemic candidaemia requiring treatment. Which is the most appropriate antifungal therapy?

a. Voriconazole.
b. Amphotericin B.
c. Fluconazole.
d. Nystatin.
e. Caspofungin.

A49 The commonest late complication of tracheostomy is:

a.   Tracheal stenosis.
b.   Tracheo-innominate artery fistula.
c.   Tracheo-oesophageal fistula.
d.   Tracheomalacia.
e.   Localised infection.

A50 Regarding the ethics of intensive care medicine, which of the following is the least appropriate principle on which to base decisions regarding patient care?

a.   Autonomy.
b.   Non-maleficence.
c.   Utility.
d.   Paternalism.
e.   Beneficence.

Paper 3

Type 'K' questions

K51 Regarding the refeeding syndrome:

a. It occurs solely as a consequence of parenteral nutrition.
b. It develops around day 4 following reinstatement of nutrition.
c. Thiamine and B vitamins should be given prior to commencing feeding after a prolonged period of poor nutrition.
d. It is a consequence of low insulin levels.

K52 A 46-year-old man is electrocuted while repairing a roadside power cable in the rain. On arrival in the Emergency Room he is maintaining an airway, has a palpable pulse but is extending to pain and has fixed and dilated pupils. His ECG is normal. A small burn wound is found over the left forearm.

a. The neurological prognosis is hopeless.
b. A normal ECG makes ongoing cardiac problems unlikely.
c. The small entry wound makes significant tissue damage unlikely.
d. Wet skin has 50% less impedance to current flow than dry skin.

K53 A 50-year-old man is brought into the Emergency Room following a cardiac arrest in a supermarket. He received immediate bystander CPR followed by defibrillation on the arrival of the paramedics, with return of spontaneous circulation after 12 minutes. He now has fixed and dilated pupils and a GCS of 5, with flexion to painful stimulus. He is admitted to the ICU and ventilated mechanically.

a. His neurological prognosis is hopeless.
b. He should be actively cooled to 32-34°C.
c. His age has a bearing on his survival chances.
d. Patients admitted to ICU following out-of-hospital cardiac arrest have less than a 10% chance of survival to hospital discharge.

K54 Regarding the use of focused abdominal ultrasound for trauma (FAST) scanning in the emergency assessment of blunt abdominal trauma:

a. Visualisation of the pericardium is a key view.
b. Free intraperitoneal fluid volumes in excess of 500ml are reliably detected.
c. It is moderately sensitive for detecting encapsulated solid organ injury.
d. Hollow viscus injury is detected in 60-70% of cases.

K55 A 34-year-old man arrives in the Emergency Room having received a stab wound to the abdomen. On arrival he is listless and has a RR of 30 breaths per minute, HR of 130bpm and a BP of 65/40mmHg. A 3cm entry wound is visible in the epigastric area. He has a firm abdomen with guarding.

a. Chest X-ray is mandatory.
b. Complete head to toe exposure should be part of the primary survey.
c. If a focused abdominal ultrasound for trauma (FAST) scan is normal, laparotomy should be deferred.
d. A fluid bolus should be given to this patient as soon as vascular access is obtained.

K56 The following are causes of the abdominal compartment syndrome:

a. High volume crystalloid resuscitation.
b. Pancreatitis.
c. Blunt abdominal trauma.
d. Laparostomy.

K57 The following are causes of elevated protein in cerebrospinal fluid:

a. Brain tumour.
b. Seizure.
c. Bacterial meningitis.
d. Neurosyphilis.

K58 A 28-year-old man presents to the Emergency Room following a mixed overdose. His wife states that he normally takes antidepressant tablets. He has a HR of 145bpm, BP of 210/150mmHg and an axillary temperature of 39.7°C. He is extremely agitated and has muscular rigidity and clonus; no extrapyramidal features are elicited.

a. MDMA ('ecstasy') should be considered as a possible cause.
b. Benzodiazepine therapy is contraindicated for this patient.
c. Intubation and mechanical ventilation may be indicated.
d. A 5-hydroxytryptamine agonist may have a role in treatment of this patient.

K59 A 58-year-old woman is recovering on the ward following treatment with a course of ceftriaxone for community-acquired pneumonia 2 weeks previously. She becomes extremely unwell with increased abdominal distension, fever and profuse watery diarrhoea. She is tachycardic and dehydrated. An abdominal X-ray shows distended loops of large bowel (10cm diameter).

a. This condition carries a mortality of 50%.
b. Colonoscopy is the investigation of choice.
c. Initial treatment should include oral clindamycin.
d. An urgent surgical opinion should be obtained.

K60 The following interventions have been shown to reduce mortality in patients with septic shock:

a. Antithrombin III.
b. Activated protein C.
c. Anti-TNF-α antibody.
d. High dose methylprednisolone.

K61 A 37-year-old man is involved in a workplace accident where he is crushed against a wall by a forklift truck. He suffers significant abdominal injuries and is in hypovolaemic shock on arrival in the Emergency Room (ATLS® class III). During laparotomy he requires a splenectomy, but also has diffuse small vessel bleeding in the retroperitoneal space. He is transfused with 18 units of packed red cells prior to transfer to the ICU and requires a further six units over the next 2 hours. Blood tests include: haematocrit 23%, platelets 30×10^9/L, fibrinogen 0.4g/L, INR 6.2.

a. Recombinant factor VIIa should be given immediately.
b. Class III shock implies blood loss of over 2L.
c. It is not mandatory to give vitamin K immediately.
d. His temperature should be checked.

K62 A 41-year-old man is involved in a car crash, and is in shock on arrival in hospital. The pelvis is unstable on 'springing' and a disrupted pelvic ring is seen on X-ray. No chest injuries are apparent clinically or radiographically. The patient is intubated and transferred to the operating theatre, and remains in shock despite fluid resuscitation with 3L crystalloid and 1L gelofusine. Initial bloods in theatre include: haematocrit 28% and a prothrombin time of 28s.

a. The presence of a coagulopathy worsens the prognosis.
b. Haematocrit is an insensitive indicator of the need for surgical intervention.
c. A high level of PEEP should be used in theatre to prevent lung de-recruitment.
d. Immediate mechanical stabilization of the pelvic ring is indicated.

K63 A 76-year-old man is trapped in a house fire and is brought to hospital 4 hours later following a difficult extrication. He requires intubation and ventilation for deteriorating gas exchange. He has burns across his entire torso anteriorly, his face, and the backs of both arms. Carbonaceous sputum is suctioned from the endotracheal tube post-intubation.

a. He has burns to approximately 45% of his body surface area.
b. A reasonable fluid regime would be 4ml/kg/% body surface area burns over the next 24 hours.
c. Use of suxamethonium would be dangerous in this situation.
d. Oxygen therapy should be titrated initially to maintain an arterial blood gas PaO_2 of around 10kPa (76mmHg).

K64 A 44-year old man is admitted to the ICU with a hospital-acquired pneumonia. Sputum and blood cultures are obtained which are positive for extended spectrum ß-lactamase(ESBL)-producing *Klebsiella pneumoniae*. The following would be appropriate empirical choices of antibiotic therapy:

a. Cefotaxime and gentamicin.
b. Piperacillin/tazobactam.
c. Imipenem.
d. Ciprofloxacin.

K65 A 66-year-old man is admitted to the ICU with chest pain and shortness of breath. Chest X-ray shows pulmonary oedema. He requires intubation and mechanical ventilation. His observations include: BP 185/120mmHg, HR 115bpm, SpO$_2$ 92% on 80% inspired O$_2$. An oesophageal Doppler probe is sited, and gives the following information: flow time corrected (FTc) 270ms, peak velocity 35cm/s, stroke volume 40ml. A fluid challenge of 250ml colloid is given over 10 minutes. Repeat readings are: FTc 275ms, peak velocity 33cm/s, stroke volume 39ml.

a. A further fluid bolus should be given.
b. A nitrate infusion is appropriate.
c. Frusemide is appropriate.
d. Cardiac contractility is normal for a man of this age.

K66 Regarding the arterial pressure wave in the hypovolaemic mechanically ventilated patient:

a. Changes in pulse pressure across the respiratory cycle better reflect hypovolaemia than changes in systolic pressure.
b. Pulse pressure is inversely proportional to stroke volume.
c. The maximum fall in systolic pressure coincides temporally with the peak inspiratory pressure.
d. The arterial pressure waveform is an unreliable guide to fluid requirement in arrhythmias.

K67 Regarding the physics of direct arterial blood pressure measurement:

a. The catheter connecting the arterial cannula to the transducer should be short, stiff and narrow to reduce resonance.
b. Bubbles and clots cause damping.
c. The resonant frequency of the system should be greater than 30Hz.
d. The primary harmonic of the system is 100Hz.

K68 Regarding the assessment of sedation on the ICU:

a. A score of 3-4 is desirable on the Richmond agitation and sedation scale.
b. The commonest form of delirium in the ICU patient is characterised by hyperarousal and agitation.
c. The Ramsay scale does not assess patient agitation.
d. The Glasgow Coma Scale is not useful for the assessment of sedation.

K69 Effects of excessive heparinisation of an arterial blood gas sample on the measured values may include:

a. Elevated $PaCO_2$.
b. Reduced $PaCO_2$.
c. Elevated PaO_2.
d. Reduced bicarbonate.

K70 A 48-year-old homeless man is brought into hospital having been found unresponsive on the street overnight. On examination he has signs of malnutrition. His observations include a temperature of 28°C, HR of 42bpm and a GCS of 5.

a. Passive re-warming should be commenced limiting temperature rise to 1°C per hour.
b. Intubation should be avoided as it may cause ventricular fibrillation.
c. Intravenous thiamine should be administered urgently.
d. If ventricular fibrillation occurs, DC cardioversion should not be attempted until the core temperature is above 30°C.

K71 The nurses ask you to review a patient on the high dependency unit who has been acting strangely. He is normally a nursing home resident and now appears agitated and confused. The following features favour a diagnosis of delirium as opposed to dementia:

a. Global cognitive impairment.
b. An insidious onset of symptoms.
c. Inattention.
d. Psychotic symptoms.

K72 Regarding acute epiglottitis in adults:

a. It is more common than in children.
b. *Haemophilus influenzae* has been largely eradicated as a cause.
c. Amoxycillin with clavulanic acid is appropriate empirical therapy.
d. Patients usually appear systemically well.

K73 A 75-year-old man is ventilated on the ICU following evacuation of a subdural haematoma 6 days previously. He develops a massive pulmonary embolism confirmed by contrast CT pulmonary arteriography. Placement of a vena cava filter is considered.

a. Thrombolysis is absolutely contraindicated.
b. Once placed the filter cannot safely be removed.
c. Vena cava filters are effective in reducing the incidence of further pulmonary emboli.
d. Vena cava filters do not improve survival.

K74 A 28-year-old man with a severe head injury is ventilated on your ICU following evacuation of a subdural haematoma. You are called because his intracranial pressure has been steadily climbing and is now 40mmHg. Appropriate treatments to buy time while awaiting a CT brain scan include:

a. Dobutamine infusion.
b. Frusemide.
c. Hyperventilation to a $PaCO_2$ of 3.5kPa (27mmHg).
d. Thiopentone bolus.

K75 The following capnograph trace on a ventilated patient is consistent with:

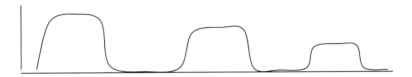

a. Endobronchial intubation following patient repositioning.
b. Air embolism.
c. Incipient cardiac arrest.
d. Bronchospasm.

K76 A 75-year-old lady presents 5 days following an anterior myocardial infarction with shortness of breath. A chest X-ray shows pulmonary venous congestion. The neck veins are distended. A systolic murmur is audible on auscultation. BP is 80/65mmHg. A pulmonary artery catheter is inserted and provides the following data: pulmonary artery oxygen saturation 88%, pulmonary artery pressure 50/23mmHg. The following are true:

a. This lady probably has papillary muscle rupture.
b. This lady is likely to need urgent surgery.
c. Electrocardiogram is the key investigation.
d. Urgent needle thoracocentesis is the treatment of choice.

K77 A 55-year-old man presents to the Emergency Room with massive haemoptysis. A history of several minor episodes of haemoptysis over the last few months is noted. He has expectorated around 500ml blood over a 3-hour period. He has a BP of 90/70mmHg, a HR of 100bpm and an SpO_2 of 85% on 15L/min oxygen via a non-rebreathing mask. You are called to assist with his management.

a. Intravenous access and rapid fluid challenge is the first priority.
b. A double-lumen tube is mandatory if tracheal intubation is required.
c. Fibreoptic bronchoscopy may be useful in this case.
d. If a bleeding source is lateralised, the patient should be ventilated with that side dependent.

K78 The following therapeutic manoeuvres improve survival in the acute respiratory distress syndrome (ARDS):

a. High levels of positive end-expiratory pressure (PEEP) >15cm H_2O.
b. Proning for >8 hours per day.
c. Low tidal volume ventilation (6ml/kg predicted body weight).
d. Alveolar recruitment manoeuvres.

K79 Regarding atrial fibrillation in the postoperative period:

a. Overall incidence is low (<1%) in non-cardiothoracic surgery.
b. It most commonly occurs in the first 3 postoperative days.
c. It resolves spontaneously in most patients.
d. It occurs in 80-90% of patients following coronary artery bypass grafting.

K80 A 67-year-old man is admitted to the coronary care unit with central chest pain. It feels like his usual angina but more severe. The pain came on at rest and has lasted for 3 hours. The ECG shows 1mm ST depression in the lateral leads. His observations are within normal limits. Creatine kinase levels were normal on admission.

a. A diagnosis of acute coronary syndrome can be made.
b. Aspirin and clopidogrel should be administered.
c. A glycoprotein IIb/IIIa inhibitor is not indicated.
d. Percutaneous coronary intervention is only beneficial in the presence of ST segment elevation.

K81 A 66-year-old man on the coronary care unit develops severe cardiogenic shock. His ECG shows significant ST-depression in the anterior leads. On examination he is cold and clammy with a BP of 80/60mmHg, HR of 120bpm (sinus tachycardia) and unrecordable oxygen saturations. Chest X-ray confirms florid pulmonary oedema. Despite appropriate inotropic support his condition fails to improve over the next few hours and an intensive care opinion is sought.

a. Myocardial infarction is the commonest cause of cardiogenic shock.
b. Mechanical ventilation is contraindicated as it will further impair cardiac output.
c. Continuous positive airway pressure (CPAP) decreases preload.
d. CPAP decreases afterload.

K82 A 49-year-old woman develops painful left-sided ophthalmoplegia following a recent bout of sinusitis. On examination she has a painful left eye with slight proptosis. Eye movement is limited in all directions, and visual acuity is reduced. A diagnosis of cavernous sinus thrombosis is considered.

a. CT brain scan is likely to be a useful investigation in this case.
b. Intravenous empirical antibiotics are indicated.
c. Mortality is 80-100%.
d. Cavernous sinus thrombosis is the commonest form of cerebral venous sinus thrombosis.

K83 The following are risk factors for the development of critical illness polyneuromyopathy:

a. Sepsis.
b. Corticosteroids.
c. Neuromuscular blocking agents.
d. Poor glycaemic control.

K84 Regarding urinalysis:

a. Red cell casts are always pathological.
b. A negative nitrite dipstick effectively excludes the presence of bacteria in the urine.
c. Hyaline casts are suggestive of bacterial endocarditis.
d. White cell casts are a normal finding.

K85 Regarding pharmacological prophylaxis of stress ulceration in the ICU:

a. Sucralfate neutralises gastric pH.
b. Proton pump inhibitors are superior to H_2-receptor antagonists in preventing clinically significant bleeding.
c. Tolerance occurs to ranitidine.
d. Antacids are effective with twice-daily dosing.

K86 A 74-year-old man is being treated on the ICU for biliary tract sepsis. Over a period of 3 days he develops marked abdominal distension. Plain radiography shows dilatation of the large bowel. The following features favour a diagnosis of acute intestinal pseudo-obstruction over mechanical obstruction:

a. The presence of air in the rectosigmoid colon on plain radiography.
b. A maximum colonic diameter of 10cm on plain radiography.
c. Free passage of contrast during a contrast enema study.
d. The presence of bowel sounds on auscultation.

K87 Renal failure may cause alterations in the following pharmacokinetic properties of a drug:

a. Absorption.
b. Distribution.
c. Metabolism.
d. Excretion.

K88 A patient with liver cirrhosis develops a major upper gastrointestinal haemorrhage due to oesophageal varices and is admitted to the ICU for resuscitation. Effective acute pharmacological management might include:

a. Glypressin.
b. Propranolol.
c. Somatostatin.
d. Isosorbide mononitrate.

K89 A 65-year-old woman is admitted to the ICU following an exploratory laparotomy and right hemicolectomy. With regard to her nutrition:

a. Parenteral feeding should be instituted only if enteral feeding has been unsuccessful over a 72-hour period.
b. Mortality is 20% higher in parenterally fed ICU patients compared with enteral feeding.
c. Delayed feeding is associated with poorer ICU outcome.
d. Parenteral feeding is associated with a higher risk of infectious complications.

K90 The following are elements of the 24-hour sepsis management bundle as advocated by the Surviving Sepsis Campaign group:

a. Administration of recombinant human activated protein C for eligible patients.
b. Methylprednisolone 1g q.d.s. for patients requiring vasopressors.
c. Maintain glucose <12.4mmol/L (225mg/dL).
d. Maintain a plateau pressure of <30cmH$_2$O for mechanically ventilated patients.

K91 A septic patient on the ICU is being assessed for suitability for recombinant activated protein C therapy. Which of the following provides supporting evidence of organ dysfunction according to the Sequential Organ Failure Assessment (SOFA) scoring system?

a. Glasgow Coma Score of <15.
b. The use of a noradrenaline infusion.
c. An International Normalised Ratio (INR) of >2.
d. A serum creatinine of >106μmol/L (>1.2mg/dL).

K92 Regarding high frequency oscillatory ventilation (HFOV):

a. Oxygenation can be improved by increasing the mean airway pressure.
b. Expiration is passive.
c. Frequency of ventilation is typically 50-100 breaths per minute.
d. CO_2 elimination can be increased by reducing the frequency of ventilation.

K93 The following forms of shock may be present in amniotic fluid embolism:

a. Distributive.
b. Cardiogenic.
c. Obstructive.
d. Haemorrhagic.

K94 Regarding non-steroidal anti-inflammatory drugs (NSAIDs) that are selective for the cyclo-oxygenase-2 (COX-2) isoenzyme:

a. They significantly reduce the risk of gastrointestinal bleeding compared with non-selective NSAIDs.
b. They cause increased thromboxane A_2 production compared with non-selective NSAIDs.
c. Rofecoxib more than doubles the risk of myocardial infarction compared with placebo.
d. They are generally less effective analgesics than non-selective NSAIDs.

K95 Regarding pharmacokinetics:

a. A half-life is half the total time taken for the drug to be completely cleared from the plasma.
b. Volume of distribution is calculated from plasma concentration x dose following an intravenous bolus of a drug.
c. Clearance is usually expressed in ml/kg/min.
d. Zero order kinetics implies enzyme saturation.

K96 The following are possible explanations for the lines A, B and C on the dose-response curve given below:

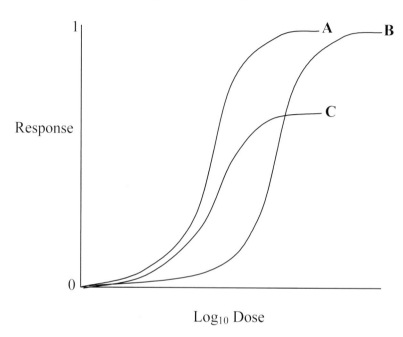

Log$_{10}$ Dose

a. A is fentanyl and B is alfentanil.
b. A is morphine and C is midazolam.
c. A is midazolam and C is midazolam in the presence of flumazenil.
d. A is morphine and C is buprenorphine.

K97 A 44-year-old man is ventilated on the ICU with abdominal sepsis. His renal function deteriorates and he requires renal replacement therapy (RRT).

a. RRT is associated with excess in-hospital mortality.
b. Acute renal failure requiring RRT is an independent risk factor for increased mortality.
c. Bleeding complications are the leading cause of death in ICU patients with acute renal failure.
d. Hospital mortality is around 15% in ICU patients requiring RRT.

K98 A patient on the ICU develops candidaemia following a prolonged period of mechanical ventilation after abdominal sepsis. C. *albicans* is isolated in blood and urine cultures. The following are likely to be effective antifungal agents:

a.   Voriconazole.
b.   Fluconazole.
c.   Caspofungin.
d.   Amphotericin B.

K99 The following are recognised complications of prone positioning in the anaesthetised patient:

a.   Stroke.
b.   Weakness of hand grip.
c.   Macroglossia.
d.   Blindness.

K100 Regarding the persistent vegetative state:

a.   Prognosis is worse if the cause is metabolic than if it is traumatic.
b.   The Glasgow Coma Scale is a useful assessment tool.
c.   Neuroimaging is usually normal.
d.   Life expectancy is normal if appropriate supportive care is provided.

Paper 3

Type 'A' answers

A1 D

A hypercalcaemic crisis is the combination of a very high blood calcium (>3.5mmol/l) and symptoms which may include nausea, lethargy, fits, coma, dehydration and renal failure. Primary hyperparathyroidism is the commonest cause, and is a cause of acute pancreatitis. Patients are very dehydrated and require extensive fluid resuscitation. Frusemide aids calciuresis and should also be given. Patients who develop renal failure will require dialysis with a calcium-free dialysate. Parathyroidectomy is increasingly a treatment of choice for patients with hypercalcaemic crisis after fluid resuscitation and lowering of serum Ca^{2+} levels. Steroids are ineffective in hypercalcaemia of malignancy but are effective in granulomatous causes such as sarcoidosis.

1. Ariyan CE, Sosa JA. Assessment and management of patients with abnormal calcium. *Crit Care Med* 2004; 32(4): s146-54.

A2 D

Hypermagnesaemia is usually a consequence of excessive iatrogenic administration. Although symptoms are non-specific, the combination of confusion, weakness, flushing and bradyarrhythmia in a patient known to be on treatment for pre-eclampsia is suggestive of this. Conduction disturbances and flaccid paralysis reflect a very high serum magnesium level of >5mmol/L (normal range 0.6-1mmol/L). Both peripartum sepsis and intracerebral haemorrhage would need to be excluded in this patient.

1. Guidelines 2000 for cardiopulmonary resuscitation and emergency cardiovascular care. Part 8: advanced challenges in resuscitation: section 1: life-threatening electrolyte abnormalities. The American Heart Association in collaboration with the International Liaison Committee on Resuscitation. *Circulation* 2000; 102(8 Suppl): I217-22.

A3   C

Hypothermia affects all body systems. Cerebral metabolic rate falls, and therefore brain oxygen consumption, which may provide relative improvement in oxygen supply to ischaemic areas of brain, as well as decreasing intracranial blood volume and improving cerebral perfusion pressure. A 'cold diuresis' may occur because of decreased reabsorption of solutes in the ascending limb of the loop of Henle. Blood glucose increases due to reduced insulin secretion from the pancreas. White cell numbers and function decrease leading to an increased incidence of sepsis including VAP, although this is more of an issue with prolonged (>24h) hypothermia. Clotting times are prolonged.

1. Bernard SA, Buist M. Induced hypothermia in critical care medicine: a review. *Crit Care Med* 2003; 31(7): 2041-51.

A4   C

The primary survey is designed to detect and address life-threatening pathology. Airway adjuncts or tracheal intubation may be required due to airway obstruction, a depressed conscious level affecting ventilation or chest injuries reducing the mechanical efficiency of breathing. Pressure should be applied to control external haemorrhage while a surgical opinion is sought. Abnormal pupillary light reflexes in conjunction with lateralising signs and a depressed conscious level suggest tentorial herniation due to diffuse axonal injury or intracerebral haematoma, and should prompt temporising measures such as mannitol, sedation and mechanical ventilation while obtaining neurosurgical advice. Percussion is a key component of chest examination and may reveal signs of haemothorax or tension pneumothorax. Although the cervical spine should be maintained in neutral alignment throughout the primary survey, a cervical spine fracture is not immediately life-threatening and should be assessed radiographically and clinically as part of the secondary survey.

1. Driscoll P, Skinner D. Initial assessment and management I: the primary survey and resuscitation. In: *ABC of Major Trauma*, 3rd Ed. Driscoll P, Skinner D, Earlam R, Eds. London: BMJ Books, 2000: 1-5.

A5   E

A penetrating abdominal injury may cause injury to vascular structures, solid organs or a hollow viscus. Peritonitis may reflect leakage of digestive tract contents from a hollow viscus and is an indication for laparotomy. The most commonly injured organs in abdominal stab wounds are the liver (40%), small bowel (30%), diaphragm (20%) and colon (15%). Chest X-ray is relatively specific for diaphragmatic injury with an abdominal stab wound, although low in sensitivity. An abdominal CT scan is the investigation of choice for assessment of injury to the liver and spleen, but lacks sensitivity for detection of mesenteric, hollow visceral and diaphragmatic injuries. A negative FAST scan has a negative predictive value for laparotomy of only 60%; it may miss free intraperitoneal blood, and will not reliably identify injuries to structures such as the diaphragm and bowel which require operative repair.

1. Udobi KF, Rodriguez A, Chiu WC, *et al.* Role of ultrasonography in penetrating abdominal trauma: a prospective clinical study. *J Trauma* 2001; 50(3): 475-9.
2. Testa PA, Legome E. (2008). Abdominal trauma, penetrating. Available: http://www.emedicine.com/emerg/TOPIC2.HTM. Last accessed 15 November 2008.

A6   E

Abdominal compartment syndrome is a combination of intra-abdominal hypertension and end-organ dysfunction, with reversal of this organ dysfunction on relief of the pressure. It generally occurs with pressures in excess of 20mmHg. Pulmonary vascular resistance increases as a result of hypoxic vasoconstriction and increased intrathoracic pressures. Lung compliance is greatly reduced and high ventilator pressures may be required. Cardiac output falls secondary to compression of venous return from the inferior vena cava and hepatic portal vein. Increased intrapleural pressure is transmitted from the abdominal compartment causing higher readings of CVP and PAOP. Renal impairment is due to a combination of factors including reduced cardiac output and increased renal venous pressure. Impaired cranial venous outflow causes a rise in intracranial pressure.

1. Bailey J, Shapiro MJ. Abdominal compartment syndrome. *Crit Care* 2000; 4: 23-9.

A7   E

The symptoms described are very non-specific and could be attributable to many disease processes. No clear history of ascending progression or antecedent viral illness is given to suggest Guillain-Barré syndrome, and no history of fatigability is given to suggest myasthenia gravis. The presence of mildly raised cerebrospinal fluid (CSF) protein, normal CSF glucose and oligoclonal bands is strongly supportive of a diagnosis of multiple sclerosis (MS). Oligoclonal bands are distinct electrophoretic patterns reflecting increased IgG production by plasma cells and are present in the CSF of 85% of patients with multiple sclerosis. They are not pathognomonic, however, being present in conditions such as systemic lupus erythematosus (SLE), neurosarcoidosis, CNS lymphoma and subacute sclerosing panencephalitis. Patients with MS may experience pseudobulbar palsy (including dysarthria) and internuclear ophthalmoplegia manifesting as occulomotor signs. A relapsing and remitting course is characteristic in the majority of cases of MS.

1. Clark CRA. Neurological disease. In: *Kumar & Clark, Clinical Medicine*, 5th Ed. Kumar PJ, Clark ML, Eds. Edinburgh: Saunders, 2002.

A8   B

NICE guidelines are available on the management of status epilepticus. Initial prehospital care includes either rectal diazepam (10-20mg) or buccal midazolam 10mg. The next stage is lorazepam 0.1mg/kg IV which may be repeated after 10-20 minutes. For established status epilepticus failing to respond to the above measures, phenytoin 15-18mg/kg IV is given at a rate not exceeding 50mg/minute (or phosphenytoin at a dose of 15-20mg phenytoin equivalents/kg). Phenobarbitone 10-15mg/kg IV may also be considered at this stage. For refractory cases, the next step is induction of general anaesthesia with propofol, midazolam or thiopentone. Phenytoin should be given at a maximum dose of 50mg/minute with cardiac monitoring. It can precipitate arrhythmias if given faster.

1. Stokes T, Shaw EJ, Juarez-Garcia A, Camosso-Stefinovic J, Baker R. Clinical guidelines and evidence review for the epilepsies: diagnosis and management in adults and children in primary and secondary care. London: Royal College of General Practitioners, 2004.
2. National Institute for Clinical Excellence. CG20 Epilepsy in adults and children: full guideline, Appendix C, 2004.

A9   C

Enteral loss of potassium and fluid may cause volume depletion, hypokalaemia and a metabolic alkalosis which carries a poor prognosis. Although these patients are often volume depleted, anaemia is usual due to blood loss per rectum with a lowered haematocrit. Leukocytosis is seen as a component of the inflammatory response. 'Left shift' refers to the fact that in severe inflammation or infection (usually bacterial), a greater proportion of immature neutrophils are present in the circulation due to excessive cytokine stimulation of the bone marrow.

1. Sheth SG. LaMont JT. Toxic megacolon. *Lancet* 1998; 351: 509-12.

A10   C

This patient has fractured ribs on CT scan, and is at risk of a tension pneumothorax. Raised intrathoracic pressure in such a case reduces venous return, reducing cardiac output and causing consequent hypotension and reflex tachycardia. While b) and d) might be reasonable in the presence of an unstable pelvic fracture with potential for massive blood loss, circulatory assessment should not take priority over airway and breathing assessment according to ATLS® teaching.

1. Advanced Trauma Life Support®, 6th Ed. American College of Surgeons, 1997.

A11   A

Raised ICP correlates with increased mortality in traumatic brain injury (TBI), and patients who respond to treatment with a fall in ICP have better outcomes. Patients with ICP monitoring *in situ* have better outcomes than historical controls, but no high quality evidence has demonstrated better outcome as a result of ICP monitoring *per se*. ICP measurement is required by definition for cerebral perfusion pressure measurement (mean arterial pressure - intracranial pressure). Haematoma requiring surgical evacuation occurs in 0.5% of cases of ICP measurement, most commonly with ventriculostomy catheter insertion. A normal CT brain scan is associated with a reduced risk of raised ICP in comatose TBI patients, but is not highly sensitive; the incidence was 13% in one series (vs.~60% with an abnormal CT).

1. Brain Trauma Foundation; American Association of Neurological Surgeons; Congress of Neurological Surgeons; Joint Section on Neurotrauma and Critical Care, AANS/CNS. Guidelines for the management of severe traumatic brain injury. VI. Indications for intracranial pressure monitoring. *J Neurotrauma* 2007; 24 Suppl 1: S65-70.

A12   B

The commonest cause of serious pelvic injury is motor vehicle accident, followed by falls from height. Mortality in patients with severe disruption of the pelvic ring is estimated at between 30%-45%, with bleeding being the major cause. Serious pelvic injury is correlated with intra-abdominal injury which should be actively excluded. Arterial embolisation may be indicated in selected cases; although most pelvic bleeding is venous, arterial embolisation may stop arterial bleeding, while fixation of the pelvic ring allows venous bleeding to tamponade itself.

1. Spahn DR, *et al*. Management of bleeding following major trauma: a European guideline. *Crit Care* 2007; 11(1): R17.

A13 B

In a patient with impending upper airway obstruction, a fibreoptic bronchoscope may occlude the narrowed airway and cause complete obstruction. An inhalational induction or rapid sequence induction are preferred techniques depending on the experience of the anaesthetist. Increased CO_2 production will be a feature of the hypermetabolic phase, and therefore minute volume will need to be increased if normocapnia is to be maintained. Morphine has a relatively slow onset and long duration of action; a shorter-acting opioid such as alfentanil is preferable. In addition, absorption kinetics of IM injections are unpredictable in such patients, and analgesia should be titrated IV. Large doses of non-depolarising relaxants may be required as burns patients are resistant to their effects from 1 week post-burn. While a warm theatre is mandatory to prevent heat losses, 37°C would be intolerable for the healthcare staff!

1.   Black RG, Kinsella J. Anaesthetic management for burns patients. *Continuing Education in Anaesthesia, Critical Care and Pain* 2001; 1(6): 177-80.

A14 C

This lady has low T3 and T4, and a raised thyroid stimulating hormone (TSH) level, all consistent with primary hypothyroidism. This may contribute to her presentation, or may be a coincidental finding. The sick euthyroid syndrome is the main differential in critically ill patients. In this syndrome patients with severe non-thyroidal illness have a low T3, low or normal T4 and a low/normal TSH, which is inappropriately low for the circulating thyroid hormone levels. In such cases there is no benefit to treatment with supplementary thyroxine/T3, as synthesis of T3 tissue receptors is upregulated maintaining a clinically euthyroid state despite biochemical evidence to the contrary.

1.   Vedig AE. Thyroid emergencies. In: *Oh's Intensive Care Manual*, 5th Ed. Bersten AD, Soni N, Eds. Edinburgh: Butterworth-Heinemann, 2003.

A15 D

The Fick principle is employed in the calculation of cardiac output using the following formula:

Cardiac output (Q) = VO_2/Arterial O_2 content - mixed venous O_2 content.

Calculation of blood oxygen content requires knowledge of the haemoglobin concentration, oxygen saturation and oxygen partial pressure using the formula (for arterial oxygen content):

$$CaO_2 = 1.39 \text{ x [Hb] x } (SaO_2/100) + 0.023 \text{ x } PaO_2$$
(Hb in g/dL, PaO_2 in kPa)

VCO_2 is not required in this example.

1. Swanevelder JLC. Cardiac physiology. In: *Fundamentals of Anaesthesia*, 2nd Ed. Pinnock C, Lin T, Smith T, Eds. London: Greenwich Medical Media, 2003.

A16 A

This patient is in shock, as demonstrated by the clinical data. The oesophageal Doppler shows a raised flow time corrected (FTc), reflecting low systemic vascular resistance [1]. A supra-normal FTc (>340ms) does not necessarily mean the patient is adequately volume loaded however. This clinical picture may be due to sepsis, vasodilator drugs or pregnancy; in this clinical context sepsis is likely. A fluid challenge should be given and the stroke volume response assessed. Peak velocity (reflecting contractility) is at the upper end of normal for this age (there is a linear decline from ≤120cm/s at 20 years old to ≤60cm/s at 90 years old). The measured flow time is reduced with increasing heart rate and a correction factor is applied to obtain FTc. In massive pulmonary embolism (a form of obstructive shock), cardiac output would be low due to impaired left ventricular filling, and FTc would be low as a result of compensatory systemic vasoconstriction to maintain blood pressure.

1. Singer M. The FTc is not an accurate marker of left ventricular preload. *Intensive Care Med* 2006; 32: 1089.

A17 A

A platinum resistance thermometer relies on the fact that resistance to current flow increases linearly with increasing temperature. A thermistor is a semiconductor composed of various metallic oxides which shows a non-linear fall in resistance with increasing temperature. A thermocouple relies on the Seebeck effect, where a small electromotive force (e.m.f) is generated at the junction of two metals which varies with temperature. This can be used to measure very high temperatures. One junction is kept at constant temperature (and e.m.f), current flow varying with the temperature of the other junction (and the potential difference between the two junctions). Radiation thermometers determine temperature based on the amount of infrared energy radiated from an object and its emissivity. This utilises Planck's law which relates the intensity of radiation from a perfect black body to temperature and wavelength. A perfect black body has an emissivity of 1, all other objects are less than 1 (the darker the object the greater the emissivity).

1.   Stoker MR. Measuring temperature. *Anaesthesia and Intensive Care Medicine* 2005; 6(6): 194-8.

A18 B

Midazolam has a short half-life when given as a bolus. However, it has an active metabolite which accumulates in renal impairment, especially in the elderly. It therefore has a long context-sensitive half-life and is not ideal. Etomidate has been shown to cause adrenal suppression and should not be used as maintenance sedation in the ICU. Clonidine is an α-2 agonist with sedative and analgesic-sparing properties. Although an attractive agent due to its lack of respiratory depression, it can cause significant hypotension and bradycardia, making it a poor choice given this patient's cardiac history. Ketamine increases intracranial pressure and is generally contraindicated in head injury management. Patients with anaphylactic egg allergy react to one of three egg proteins (ovoalbumin, ovomucoid and conalbumin) whereas the propofol lipid vehicle contains purified egg phosphatide (lecithin) which is not known to be allergenic [1]. Egg allergy is not listed in the Diprivan [proprietary formulation of propofol] product information leaflet as a contraindication to use.

1. Bradley AED, Tober KES, Brown RE. Use of propofol in patients with food allergies [letter]. *Anaesthesia* 2008; 63: 439.
2. Peck TE, Hill SA, Williams M. *Pharmacolocy for Anaesthesia and Intensive Care*, 2nd Ed. London: Greenwich Medical Media, 2003.

A19   C

The scale on the vertical axis is 0.1mV/mm. The QT interval is as stated, normally <0.44s when corrected for heart rate (QTc = QT/√R-R interval). A cardiac monitor has a typical frequency range of around 0.5-40Hz, compared with a diagnostic ECG which has a broader range (0.05-100Hz). The cardiac monitor therefore filters out high frequency interference (e.g. capacitance linkage from other equipment) and low frequency interference (e.g. respiratory motion). P-wave morphology and S-T changes are more clearly defined with the high frequency range of a diagnostic ECG machine. Lead I measures the potential difference between the right and left arms, with the left leg acting as neutral. The measured amplitude of the ECG signal is 1-2mV, whereas the true potential in the heart is around 90mV. This potential is attenuated by passage through the tissues.

1. Lee J. ECG monitoring in theatre. *Update in Anaesthesia* 2000; 11: Article 5.

A20   D

Latex allergy can present as an IgE mediated anaphylaxis. Symptoms usually occur some time (20-30 mins) following exposure, unlike drug anaphylaxis which occurs immediately following intravenous injections. It is more common in those routinely exposed to latex (e.g. healthcare workers) and those with a variety of food allergies including avocado, chestnut and kiwi. Patients with spina bifida and cerebral palsy are also at risk, probably due to repeated urinary catheterisation. Immediate management is the same as that for drug anaphylaxis; in addition all latex products should be removed. Vagal reactions may cause bronchospasm, but not tachycardia. Laryngospasm is not possible with a correctly positioned endotracheal tube. Pneumothorax might cause the same cardiovascular picture but not usually widespread bronchospasm.

1. Ballantyne JC. Latex anaphylaxis: another case, another cause. *Anesth Analg* 1995; 81: 1303-4.

A21   C

Numerous guidelines now exist regarding the management of ICU delirium. Non-pharmacological strategies include maintenance of a normal sleep-wake cycle as far as possible (lights off at night), orientation of the patient (clock on the wall), ensuring spectacles and hearing aids are available if required, and eliminating organic drivers of delirium such as pain and hypoxia. Benzodiazepines are not considered first-line therapy unless to treat a benzodiazepine or alcohol withdrawal delirium. A propofol infusion may mask the outward signs of delirium, but is likely to delay weaning time and length of ICU stay. It may be useful to gain control in an extremely agitated patient who is at risk of harming themselves or others. Haloperidol either enterally or parenterally titrated to the level of agitation is recommended, with vigilance for side effects including long Q-T syndrome, extrapyramidal signs and, rarely, the neuroleptic-malignant syndrome.

1. Chevrolet J-C, Jolliet P. Clinical review: agitation and delirium in the critically ill - significance and management. *Crit Care* 2007; 11: 214.
2. Borthwick M, *et al.* Detection, prevention and treatment of delirium in critically ill patients. United Kingdom Clinical Pharmacy Association, 2006.

A22   B

Lundberg described three types of abnormal intracranial pressure (ICP) waves found in cases of raised intracranial pressure. Type A (plateau waves) are largest in amplitude (50-100mmHg above baseline ICP) and duration (5-20 minutes). They are thought to be due to cerebral vasodilatation in response to critically low cerebral perfusion. This dilatation further raises ICP, compromising cerebral perfusion and increasing the risk of brain herniation. Type B waves have an amplitude of up to 50mmHg, and a duration of <2 minutes. They also reflect reduced intracranial compliance, but are a less sinister finding than A waves. Type C waves (also known as Hering-Traube waves) have a duration of approximately 5 minutes and an amplitude of <20mmHg. They may be pathological but can also be seen in normal individuals and are of less clinical significance than type A and B waves. Lundberg waves occur over a period of time and should not be confused with the three peaks of the normal intracranial pressure waveform seen in normal individuals and related to the arterial waveform.

1.   Ross N, Eynon CA. Intracranial pressure monitoring. *Current Anaesthesia & Critical Care* 2005; 16: 255-61.

A23   C

The appropriate investigation of suspected pulmonary embolism is influenced by the pretest probability of the condition. This can be assessed with reference to various scoring systems (e.g. the Geneva score, the Canadian Pulmonary Embolism score). Factors such as a previous history of thromboembolic disease, recent predisposing surgery, suggestive blood gas values, tachycardia and old age all increase the pretest probability. A positive D-dimer result is 96-98% sensitive, meaning that false negatives are possible though rare, and further investigation should be pursued if clinical suspicion is high. A high-probability V/Q scan in a patient without pre-existing cardiopulmonary disease is diagnostic of pulmonary embolism. If the scan is equivocal, however, further imaging should be pursued. While contrast CT may miss subsegmental emboli, false positives are rare (high specificity). An elevated troponin is often found in significant pulmonary embolism. It is not a useful diagnostic feature, but may be useful in risk stratification of patients with a confirmed diagnosis.

Table 1. Geneva score for assessing probability of pulmonary embolism.

Criterion	Value	Points
Age	60-79	+1
	80+	+2
Previous DVT/PE?	Yes	+2
Surgery in last 4 weeks	Yes	+3
Heart rate >100bpm	Yes	+1
$PaCO_2$ (mmHg)	<35	+2
	35-39	+1
PaO_2 (mmHg)	<49	+4
	49-59	+3
	60-71	+2
	71-82	+1
CXR findings	Band atelectasis	+1
	Elevated hemidiaphragm	+1

Total score: <5 low probability, 5-8 intermediate probability, >8 high probability of pulmonary embolism

1. Tapson VF. Acute pulmonary embolism. *New Engl J Med* 2008; 358(10): 1037-52.
2. Wicki J, *et al.* Assessing clinical probability of pulmonary embolism in the emergency ward: a simple score. *Arch Intern Med* 2001; 161: 92-7.

A24   E

Malignant hyperthermia is a rare disorder of calcium homeostasis in skeletal muscle caused by a defect in the ryanodine receptor. Suxamethonium and volatile anaesthetic agents can trigger excessive release of calcium ions from the sarcoplasmic reticulum causing generalised excessive muscle contraction in susceptible individuals. Masseter spasm is common but not universal. Excessive metabolic activity leads to pyrexia (temperature rise of 1-2°C/hour), metabolic acidosis, rhabdomyolysis, renal failure, hyperkalaemia, arrhythmias, hypoxia, hypercarbia, disseminated intravascular coagulation and cerebral and pulmonary oedema. Treatment involves active cooling and dantrolene administration (2-3mg/kg bolus initially followed by a further 1mg/kg bolus p.r.n., up to a maximum dose of 10mg/kg). The patient requires invasive monitoring in a critical care area. Mortality remains above 10%.

1. Association of Anaesthetists of Great Britain and Ireland. (2007). Management of a malignant hyperthermia crisis. Available: http://www.aagbi.org/publications/guidelines/docs/malignanthyp07a mended.pdf. Last accessed 20 November 2008.

A25 E

Plateau pressure is measured after a 0.5 second end-inspiratory pause. It reflects lung compliance and is distinct from peak pressure which is a measure of both compliance and resistive forces. A decelerating flow pattern will reduce peak airway pressure compared with a flat or accelerating waveform. High inspiratory flow rates will increase peak pressure but not plateau pressure if the tidal volume remains unchanged. Plateau pressure and peak pressure are both increased by increasing tidal volume, and by any condition causing reduced pulmonary compliance (pulmonary oedema, pneumothorax, ascites, etc.).

1. Grinnan DC, Truwit JD. Clinical review: respiratory mechanics in spontaneous and assisted ventilation. *Crit Care* 2005; 9(5): 472-84.

A26 E

Heparin may cause heparin-induced thrombocytopaenia by immune mechanisms. A huge number of drugs may cause thrombocytopaenia including cephalosporins, penicillins, vancomycin, linezolid, non-steroidal anti-inflammatory drugs, diuretics, anticonvulsants and tricyclic antidepressants. Opiates are not implicated.

1. British National Formulary 53. London: BMJ Publishing Group Ltd, 2007.

A27   D

Given that the deterioration coincided with mechanical ventilation, a likely explanation is progressive hyperinflation of the chest reducing venous return and compromising cardiac output. This may result from inadequate expiratory time and/or excessive tidal volume being set on the ventilator. Disconnection of the circuit would allow complete passive exhalation and should restore venous return and cardiac output. Cardiovascular deterioration is a common complication following intubation and mechanical ventilation of such patients. The clinical information suggests a vasoconstricted circulation (narrow pulse pressure), and commencing noradrenaline in such circumstances is likely to further decrease cardiac output. The propofol infusion is not set at an especially high rate, and the narrow pulse pressure and tachycardia do not suggest that oversedation is the primary issue. The clinical examination findings do not suggest tension pneumothorax.

1. Davidson AC. The pulmonary physician in critical care 11: Critical care management of respiratory failure resulting from COPD. *Thorax* 2002; 57: 1079-84.

A28   D

Pregnancy tends to improve asthma in a third of sufferers, and worsen symptoms in another third. Symptoms are usually worst between weeks 24-36, improving in the peripartum period (acute severe asthma is very rare during labour). Almost all asthma drugs can be given as normal, since the very small risks of foetal harm are outweighed by the problems of poorly controlled asthma in pregnancy, which is associated with premature birth, low birth weight and increased perinatal mortality. Methylxanthines and ß2 agonists have not been shown to be teratogenic. Prednisolone has a weak association with cleft lip and palate but should be used if necessary for symptom control. Little data are available on the use of leukotriene antagonists in pregnancy, and these should be avoided. Of the 'obstetric' drugs, syntocinon and prostaglandin E2 are safe, but prostaglandin F2a (occasionally required to stimulate uterine contraction for haemorrhage control) is a potent cause of bronchospasm and should be avoided.

1. British Thoracic Society, Scottish Intercollegiate Guidelines Network. British guideline on the management of asthma. Available online at: http://www.brit-thoracic.org.uk.

A29   A

The physiology of proning is complex and summarised in numerous reviews. In general, ventilation seems to be more homogenously distributed in the prone position. This may be due to greater compliance of the dorsal lung which is no longer compressed by the cardiac mass, decreased anterior chest wall compliance causing a relative redistribution of ventilation to the dorsal regions, and a more evenly distributed pleural pressure gradient. Perfusion is thought to remain largely dorsal in the prone position (i.e. not greatly affected by gravity). The net effect is an improvement in V/Q matching and a reduction in physiological shunt.

1. Pelosi P, *et al*. Effects of the prone position on respiratory mechanics and gas exchange during acute lung injury. *Am J Respir Crit Care Med* 1998; 157: 387-93.
2. Pelosi P, Brazzi L, Gattinoni L. Prone position in acute respiratory distress syndrome. *Eur Respir J* 2002; 20: 1017-28.

A30   C

Overall, there is no evidence to support rhythm control over rate control in terms of long-term mortality benefit. However, in a young patient with acute onset atrial fibrillation cardioversion is desirable and achievable. Digoxin, metoprolol and verapamil are all useful rate controlling drugs, but will not restore sinus rhythm. From the clinical information given, this lady has no 'high-risk' features (chest pain, critical perfusion, heart rate >150bpm), and therefore electrical cardioversion is not warranted in the first instance. Flecainide is a Vaughn-Williams class Ic antiarrhythmic agent and is an appropriate choice in a young patient with no structural heart disease.

1.   Advanced Life Support Provider Manual, 4th Ed. Resuscitation Council UK, 2004.

A31   C

Non ST-segment elevation myocardial infarction (NSTEMI) is by definition confirmed retrospectively by the presence of elevated cardiac enzymes, of which cardiac troponin is the most specific. The risk of reinfarction and cardiac death correlates with the magnitude of the rise in troponin. ST changes do not necessarily imply myocardial infarction, but the presence of 2mm ST depression in two contiguous leads on the ECG is associated with a ten-fold increase in 1-year mortality, reflecting widespread subendocardial ischaemia.

1.   Prasad A, *et al.* Current management of non-ST-segment elevation acute coronary syndrome: reconciling the results of randomized controlled trials. *Eur Heart J* 2003; 24: 1544-53.

A32   E

The left ventricle will be hypertrophied and poorly compliant, and will require a high preload and high filling pressures. The 'atrial kick' is of greater importance to help fill the stiff left ventricle, and arrhythmias such as atrial fibrillation should be aggressively cardioverted. The intra-aortic balloon pump inflates in diastole improving coronary perfusion, and deflates in ventricular systole reducing afterload. It is useful in reducing cardiac work. It is contraindicated in severe aortic regurgitation since it increases the regurgitant fraction. Maintenance of a high systemic vascular resistance is important to maintain coronary perfusion pressure. Diuretics may be used in cases of fluid overload or pulmonary oedema, but should be used with caution since a drop in preload can severely compromise cardiac output in these patients.

1.   Konstadt S. Anesthesia for non-cardiac surgery in the patient with cardiac disease. *Can J Anaesth* 2005; 52(6): R1-3.

A33   C

Cerebral venous sinus thrombosis may prevent in various ways. Headache which may be insidious in onset and progressive in nature is present in 80%. Occlusion of the cerebral venous drainage (most commonly the superior sagittal sinus and the lateral sinuses) develops over a period of days or weeks, allowing collateral flow to develop which may account for the slow onset of symptoms. Haemorrhagic infarction of the cortex and adjacent white matter may complicate the picture. Signs include ophthalmoplegia, focal neurological deficits, drowsiness and fits. A contrast CT brain scan may show the classic (but subtle) 'empty delta sign' where a triangular area of enhancement is seen on multiple contiguous transverse CT images in the region of the superior sagittal sinus. However, a CT scan is entirely normal in 10-20% of cases. Magnetic resonance venography is the imaging technique of choice. The condition is more likely in young women, especially in the puerperium, and is also associated with any hypercoagulable state (this woman has a previous miscarriage which could be relevant). Systemic or localised infections may also precipitate the condition. Therapeutic anticoagulation is indicated even in the presence of venous infarction; when treated appropriately, 57-86% of patients make a full functional recovery.

1.   Allroggen H, Abbott RJ. Cerebral venous sinus thrombosis. *Postgrad Med J* 2000; 76: 12-5.

A34   D

Critical illness polyneuromyopathy (CIP) is a common cause of weakness in the ICU patient, and is especially prevalent in patients ventilated for more than a week. Other causes must be considered, however, with a careful history, examination and further tests where indicated. The mnemonic 'MUSCLES' may be of value in assessing such patients:

- **M**edications.
- **U**ndiagnosed neuromuscular conditions.
- **S**pinal cord disease.
- **C**ritical illness polyneuromyopathy.
- **L**oss of muscle mass.
- **E**lectrolyte disorders.
- **S**ystemic disease.

A flaccid quadriparesis is a common presentation of CIP, but extensor plantars and hyperreflexia should raise suspicion of an upper motor neurone problem, and necessitates urgent imaging of the brain and spinal cord. Serum creatinine kinase is elevated in 50% of cases of critical illness myopathy. Four equal twitches is a normal response to train-of-four nerve stimulation. If fade or a reduced count is present this should raise suspicion of residual neuromuscular blockade.

1. Maramattom BV, Wijdicks EFM. Acute neuromuscular weakness in the intensive care unit. *Crit Care Med*; 34(11): 2835-41.

A35 E

Diagnosis of clinically significant urinary tract infection in the catheterised ICU patient is difficult and must be based on the clinical picture as well as microbiological evidence. Candida isolated from urine is a common finding in ICU patients. In general this does not require treatment unless isolated from multiple sites, although treatment should be considered if high levels are present ($>10^4$cfu/ml), signs of infection are present, and no other source of infection is apparent. Pyuria is defined as >10 white blood cells/μl urine. In isolation it does not mandate antimicrobial treatment, although it should prompt a search for urinary pathogens. Non-infectious causes of pyuria include recent antibiotic treatment, systemic inflammatory conditions, nephrolithiasis and drugs including corticosteroids. A urine culture $>10^3$cfu/mL bacteria mandates antibiotic therapy only in the presence of clinical indicators of infection, and may represent simple colonisation if such indicators are absent. While a positive nitrite and leukocyte esterase on dipstick testing mandates further investigation, it is not sufficiently specific to justify antibiotic treatment in the absence of supporting evidence of urinary tract infection.

1. Calandra T, Cohen J for the International Sepsis Forum Definition of Infection in the ICU. The International Sepsis Forum Consensus Conference on Definitions of Infection in the Intensive Care Unit. *Crit Care Med* 2005; 33(7): 1538-48.

A36   B

The Budd-Chiari syndrome is caused by occlusion of the hepatic venous outflow by a variety of conditions including inherited thrombophilias, use of the oral contraceptive pill, pregnancy, chronic inflammatory conditions and various tumours. It may present acutely with the classic triad of ascites, hepatomegaly and abdominal pain, or may present insidiously. In the latter case, a collateral circulation has time to develop and ascites may be minimal. Doppler ultrasonography is a reasonably sensitive and specific screening investigation, but the gold standard is hepatic venography. Management of the Budd-Chiari syndrome includes medical treatment of ascites (diuretics, sodium restriction), anticoagulation and reduction of the venous pressure which may require a portosystemic shunt. The serum-ascites albumin gradient differentiates between portal hypertensive ascites (>1.1) and other causes, and is considered more accurate than the older classification of exudates and transudates based on ascitic fluid protein concentration. Nephrotic syndrome can cause ascites and peripheral oedema, but is defined as a urine protein excretion of >3g/day. Spontaneous bacterial peritonitis is likely if a neutrophil count of >250/mm^3 is found in the ascitic fluid sample.

1. Chung RT, *et al.* Case 15-2006: a 46-year-old woman with sudden onset of abdominal distention. *N Engl J Med* 2006; 354: 2166-75.

A37 D

Ischaemic hepatitis is characterised by a marked elevation in aminotransferase levels in the absence of other causes. It is thought to be caused by hepatocyte hypoxia secondary to a period of profound hypotension. Patients with cardiac failure causing hepatic venous congestion seem to be at much greater risk. The histological hallmark of the condition is centrilobular necrosis. In addition to raised AST and ALT, lactate dehydrogenase is also typically elevated, as is the prothrombin time. Mild elevation of bilirubin is also common. Acalculous cholecystitis and ICU jaundice are not associated with dramatic elevation of transaminases, and ultrasound abnormalities of the gallbladder wall are usual with the former.

1. Seeto RK, Fenn B, Rockey DC. Ischemic hepatitis: clinical presentation and pathogenesis. *Am J Med* 2000; 109: 109-13.

A38 D

Tazocin is largely excreted unchanged in the urine. Dose should be dropped from t.d.s. to b.d. in severe renal impairment. Dose adjustments are required for most antibiotics except metronidazole and macrolides. Digoxin is excreted unchanged in the urine; the terminal elimination half-life is 30-40 hours with normal renal function, rising to 100 hours in patients with severe renal impairment. Atenolol is eliminated by renal excretion and requires dose adjustment in severe renal impairment. Metformin is also excreted unchanged in the urine and may cause hypoglycaemia if given in severe renal impairment. Amiodarone has a long terminal elimination half-life (25 days). It is metabolised by the cytochrome P450 CYP34A family to N-desethylamiodarone, which may have some antiarrhythmic effect. Both the parent compound and metabolite are excreted almost completely in bile and no dose adjustment is required in renal impairment.

1. [Product data sheets].

A39 E

Numerous markers of malnutrition are available, but in the absence of a gold standard test their validity in the critically ill patient is questionable. Hepatic secretory proteins such as albumin are markers of visceral protein stores. However, the half-life of albumin is 18 days. In addition, several factors affect hepatic albumin synthesis apart from malnutrition, such as the systemic inflammatory response and/or acute infection. Anthropometric measurements such as triceps skin fold thickness are standardised but not validated in ICU patients. A loss of >10% ideal body weight is a specific indicator of malnutrition, but most critically ill patients develop oedema which masks such a drop in weight. The creatinine height index estimates lean body mass from a 24-hour urinary creatinine assay compared with standard values for a given height. It is influenced by factors such as systemic stress and renal impairment, both common in ICU patients.

1.   Cerra FB, et al. Applied nutrition in ICU patients: a consensus statement of the American College of Chest Physicians. Chest 1997; 111: 769-78.

A40 D

Cocaine is an indirectly acting sympathomimetic drug which may cause hypertensive crises due to reduced reuptake of noradrenaline at sympathetic nerve terminals. The mainstay of treatment is administration of a benzodiazepine which ameliorates both the cerebral and cardiovascular manifestations of cocaine toxicity. If blood pressure control is required despite such therapy, alpha-blockade is preferable to beta-blockade; the latter may increase the blood pressure due to unopposed alpha stimulation.

1.   Ghuran A, Nolan J. Recreational drug misuse: issues for the cardiologist. Heart 2000; 83: 627-33.

A41 D

Gamma-hydroxybutyrate (GHB) is an increasingly popular recreational drug, and is also a muscle-bulking agent used by bodybuilders. It is derived from gamma-hydroxybutyric acid (GABA) and induces a state of euphoria when taken in small doses. Features of toxicity include hypothermia, bradycardia, reduced conscious level, respiratory acidosis and emesis. Patients may require intubation to protect the airway and normalise gas exchange for a short period of time; the effects of overdose usually wear off after several hours. A typical case of GHB overdose is one of respiratory depression interspersed with periods of violent agitation provoked by stimulation. Serious harm is unusual provided the airway is protected, and management is supportive. Evidence of trauma or other drug ingestion should be sought. Ecstasy poisoning is characterised by tachycardia and hyperpyrexia. Phencyclidine is a hallucinogen which induces a dissociative state and may cause coma in overdose, but hypertension, nystagmus, salivation, bronchorrhoea are characteristic findings. Ketamine is a dissociative anaesthetic and recreational drug of abuse which causes loss of awareness with preservation of airway and cardiovascular reflexes. It causes hypertension and increases heart rate in large doses. A pure heroin overdose would respond to naloxone.

1. Mason PE, Kerns WP. Gamma hydroxybutyric acid (GHB) intoxication. *Acad Emerg Med* 2002; 9(7): 730-9.

A42 B

High frequency oscillatory ventilation (HFOV) delivers small tidal volumes at an extremely high frequency (from 3-15Hz). Despite the fact that tidal volumes are typically 1-3ml/kg, less than the physiological dead space, gas exchange is effected by a variety of mechanisms including direct bulk flow, pendelluft, cardiogenic mixing and molecular diffusion [1]. When used in patients with acute respiratory distress syndrome (ARDS), oxygenation typically improves although elimination of CO_2 is modestly reduced. The frequency, I:E ratio, driving pressure and mean airway pressure are all set by the clinician; the tidal volume is provided by oscillations of pressure around the mean value (delta P). This is directly related to the driving pressure, and inversely related to the frequency.

1. Krishnan JA, Brower RG. High-frequency ventilation for acute lung injury and ARDS. *Chest* 2000; 118: 795-807.

A43 C

The syndrome of haemolysis, elevated liver enzymes and low platelets (HELLP) is commonly associated with hypertensive disease of pregnancy, and is present in 4-12% of cases of pre-eclampsia. However, 20% of cases of HELLP have no antecedent history of hypertension or proteinuria. The pathogenesis is poorly understood and may overlap with pre-eclampsia. The ensuing systemic microvascular injury causes microangiopathic haemolytic anaemia, thrombocytopenia and periportal hepatic necrosis. Haemolysis is reflected on the blood film as fragmented red cells (schistocytes) and in a raised lactate dehydrogenase and unconjugated bilirubin. The condition is clinically similar to the acute fatty liver of pregnancy (AFLP), but hypoglycaemia, prolonged prothrombin time and progression to acute hepatic failure are uncommon in HELLP. The mainstay of treatment is delivery of the foetus. Corticosteroids do not improve mortality but are useful since they improve clinical and laboratory parameters and delay the need for induction of labour. This buys time for foetal lung maturation.

1. Mihu D, *et al.* HELLP syndrome - a multisystemic disorder. *J Gastrointestin Liver Dis* 2007; 16(4): 419-24.

A44 B

Aspirin in a low dose selectively inhibits platelet cyclo-oxygenase, reducing thromboxane A$_2$ production and platelet aggregation. Vessel wall epoprostanol (prostacyclin) production (which opposes platelet aggregation and enhances vasodilatation) is unaffected. Even in high doses aspirin is a less effective analgesic agent than most non-steroidal anti-inflammatory drugs. Aspirin irreversibly inhibits cyclo-oxygenase, and its antiplatelet effects are terminated only with the synthesis of new platelets. All NSAIDs can displace warfarin from its albumin binding site, promoting anticoagulation. Haemodialysis is a useful treatment for enhancing elimination of aspirin in overdose since a significant proportion is not protein bound (30%).

1. Analgesics. In: *Pharmacology for Anaesthesia and Intensive Care,* 2nd Ed. Peck TE, Hill SA, Williams M. London: Greenwich Medical Media, 2003: 139-48.

A45   B

The hepatic extraction ratio is the fraction of the drug entering the liver in the blood which is extracted during one pass of the blood through the liver. This can range from 0 to 100%. Drugs such as midazolam have a high extraction ratio. Since there are plenty of enzymes to metabolise such drugs as they pass through the liver, increasing the blood flow through the liver will increase hepatic clearance of the drug. Metabolism of such drugs is therefore 'flow-limited'. Drugs such as phenytoin have a low extraction ratio reflecting a paucity of enzymes available to metabolise the drug. For such drugs, increasing liver blood flow will not significantly increase hepatic extraction, since the enzyme system is working to maximum capacity already; more drug will simply 'bypass' this system if flow is increased. Such drugs are 'metabolism-limited'. Drugs with a high hepatic extraction ratio have low bioavailability since first pass metabolism is high.

1. Smith TC. Pharmacokinetics. In: *Fundamentals of Anaesthesia*, 2nd Ed. Pinnock C, Lin T, Smith T, Eds. London: Greenwich Medical Media, 2003: 573-86.

A46   B

Sickle cell disease is characterised by an abnormal haemoglobin (HbS) in which an amino acid substitution on the beta-chain renders haemoglobin susceptible to sickling in conditions of acidosis, hypothermia, hypoxia and stress. The principles of peri-operative care include adequate hydration, maintenance of normothermia, correction of acidosis, excellent analgesia and avoidance of hypoxaemia. Exchange transfusion may be appropriate before major surgery to HbS levels of <30%, although this is not routinely indicated and should be based on consultation with a haematologist.

1. Haxby E, Flynn F, Bateman C. Anaesthesia for patients with sickle cell disease or other haemoglobinopathies. *Anaesthesia and Intensive Care Medicine* 2007; 8(5): 217-9.

A47   B

Clostridium difficile infection may be caused by one of over 150 different strains (ribotypes). In recent years the incidence of infection with ribotype 027 is increasing; this form is more virulent due to prolonged production of the exotoxins responsible for symptoms. For uncomplicated cases oral metronidazole is the treatment of choice since it is generally effective and cheap. In addition, the antibiotic associated with the outbreak should be stopped if possible; quinolones, clindamycin and cephalosporins all increase the risk of *C. difficile* infection dramatically. If an ileus is present oral administration of either metronidazole or vancomycin will be ineffective. Intravenous vancomycin is of no use since it does not penetrate the large bowel in sufficient dose. Intravenous metronidazole is effective, however, and is the treatment of choice for this patient. Probiotics have a weak evidence base and are not currently recommended for the treatment of this condition. Intravenous pooled human immunoglobulin has been shown to be effective in small case series for treatment-refractory cases, and may be an option if antibiotic therapy is unsuccessful. It is not a first-line treatment however.

1.   Kuijper EJ, van Dissel JT, Wilcox MH. *Clostridium difficile*: changing epidemiology and new treatment options. *Current Opinion in Infectious Diseases* 2007; 20: 376-83.

A48   E

Voriconazole may cause QT prolongation in susceptible individuals, and should be avoided in the presence of other risk factors for long-QT syndrome; this patient is on amiodarone which also prolongs the QT interval. Amphotericin B has a wide spectrum of activity and is effective against most Candida species, but it has a significant risk of renal impairment and should not be first-line treatment in a man with precarious renal function. Fluconazole is effective against *C. albicans* but less so against other forms of Candida including *C. glabrata* which is resistant in 60% of cases [1]. Since the species is not stated, fluconazole may not be suitable in this case. Nystatin is used in the treatment of *C. albicans* infection of the skin and mucous membranes, but is not suitable for systemic candidiasis in a critically ill patient. Caspofungin has a broad spectrum of activity and is suitable for the treatment of invasive Candida and Aspergillus infections.

1. Odds FC, *et al.* One year prospective survey of Candida bloodstream infections in Scotland. *Journal of Medical Microbiology* 2007; 56: 1066-75.
2. British Medical Association. British National Formulary. London: BMJ Publishing, 2007: 317-23.

A49 A

Tracheal stenosis is the commonest late complication of tracheostomy. Narrowing of the tracheal lumen occurs most commonly at the level of the stoma or directly above it. Some patients may have stenosis more caudally at the site of the tracheostomy tube cuff or distal tip. Commonly, granulation tissue develops as a result of bacterial infection and chondritis which weakens the anterior and lateral tracheal walls. Subsequent fibrosis and stenosis then occur. In other cases tracheal wall ischaemia may be the precipitating insult for granulation tissue formation. The overall incidence of tracheal stenosis may be high (31% of patients had >10% stenosis in one bronchoscopic study following percutaneous tracheostomy), but clinically significant stenosis requiring intervention occurs in 3-12% of patients. Risk factors include prolonged transtracheal intubation prior to stoma creation, stomal site infection, old age, sepsis, oversized cannulae, excessive tube motion and prolonged placement. Patients may be asymptomatic until 75% airway narrowing has occurred; cough and inability to clear secretions, exertional dyspnoea and stridor may all occur with increasing degree of stenosis. Since symptoms are non-specific, a high index of clinical suspicion is required. A tracheo-innominate artery fistula is a rare but almost universally fatal complication of tracheostomy. The innominate artery crosses the trachea at the level of the ninth tracheal ring, and therefore risk is increased with a low cannula placement. Most cases occur within 3-4 weeks, with bleeding, massive haemoptysis and near-100% mortality. Tracheo-oesophageal fistula occurs in <1% of cases, and is more commonly seen with injury to the posterior tracheal wall during tracheostomy. Excessive secretion production and recurrent aspiration may suggest this complication. Tracheomalacia is a result of ischaemic injury to the trachea followed by chondritis and subsequent destruction and necrosis of supporting tracheal cartilage. As with tracheal stenosis, symptoms may be non-specific. Flow-volume loops may show a variable intrathoracic obstruction (expiratory collapse of the trachea). Localised infection is usually an early complication of tracheostomy.

1.   Epstein SK. Late complications of tracheostomy. *Respir Care* 2005; 50(4): 542-9.

A50   D

Autonomy means respect for the patient's wishes and attitudes regarding the treatment they wish to receive. Non-maleficence is the duty of the physician not to do harm to the patient or members of the healthcare team or wider community. Benificence reflects the duty of the healthcare team to 'do good' to the patient by effecting a cure, relieving suffering and generally acting in their best interests. Utility is the principle of doing the greatest good for the greatest number of patients with the resources available; it may also be viewed as the obligation to provide a net balance of benefits over harms with limited resources, and is considered a subset of beneficence by some authors. Justice is the obligation to distribute benefits and harms fairly. Paternalism implies that 'the doctor knows best' for the patient. While this may be true in some contexts (e.g. which antibiotic is the appropriate treatment for the patient's infection), in the wider sense it contradicts the principle of patient autonomy. The physician has a duty to act as the patient would wish him to act rather than imposing his own beliefs. Giving a blood transfusion to a devout Jehovah's Witness would be an extreme example of paternalism.

1.   Oh TE. Ethics in intensive care. In: *Oh's Intensive Care Manual*, 5th Ed. Bersten AD, Soni N, Eds. Edinburgh: Butterworth-Heinemann, 2003.
2.   Childress JF. The normative principles of medical ethics. In: *Medical Ethics*, 2nd Ed. Veatch RM. London: Jones & Bartlett, 1997: 29-56.

Paper 3

Type 'K' answers

K51   FTTF

The refeeding syndrome occurs with both enteral and parenteral nutrition, and usually becomes apparent 3-4 days from the beginning of nutrition. These patients are at risk of Wernicke's encephalopathy, and prophylactic thiamine and B vitamin complex should be given. Depletion of adenosine triphosphate (ATP) with hypophosphataemia can lead to haemolytic anaemia, leukocyte dysfunction and platelet abnormalities. Problems stem from the sudden increase in insulin in response to the switch from starvation to carbohydrate metabolism. The insulin causes cellular uptake of phosphate and consequent hypophosphataemia.

1.   Fung AT, Rimmer J. Hypophosphataemia secondary to oral refeeding syndrome in a patient with long-term alcohol misuse. *MJA* 2005; 183(6): 324-6.

K52   FTFF

The initial assessment of pupils may be misleading and good recovery has been reported despite the initial presence of apparently hopeless neurological signs. A large case series has demonstrated that in the presence of a normal ECG it is unlikely that cardiac problems will develop later. Small electrical burn entry wounds can be associated with massive muscle damage and rhabdomyolysis; early surgical exploration and debridement is indicated if deep muscle injury is suspected. Wet skin has an impedance of around 100 times less than dry skin, allowing a much greater current to flow for a given voltage with consequently greater tissue damage.

1.   Soni N. Electrical injury. *Current Anaesthesia & Critical Care* 2002; 13: 92-6.

K53   FTTF

Initial neurological presentation is a poor predictor of outcome following return of spontaneous circulation (ROSC) post-arrest. 4% of patients with fixed dilated pupils during the first 24h subsequently recover good neurological function, and attempts to predict return of neurological function are considered unreliable in the first 72h post-ROSC. Age has a modest adverse effect on outcome. The overall survival rate for out-of-hospital cardiac arrest patients ventilated in the ICU is around 30%; in the over 80-year age group, this falls to 18.8% so the decision to admit cannot be based solely on age. Two prospective randomised controlled trials have demonstrated improved survival rates for out-of-hospital cardiac arrest patients treated with mild-moderate hypothermia (32-34°C) for 12-24 hours. Such cooling should be instituted as quickly as possible.

1.   Nolan JP, *et al*. Outcome following admission to UK intensive care units after cardiac arrest: a secondary analysis of the ICNARC Case Mix Programme Database. *Anaesthesia* 2007; 62: 1207-16.

K54   TTTF

FAST scanning involves ultrasound viewing of the pericardial space (subxiphoid view), the splenorenal and hepatorenal spaces, the paracolic gutters and the pouch of Douglas. It can reliably detect free intraperitoneal fluid if the volume present is >500ml. Although operator-dependent, a basic level of skill can rapidly be acquired by novices with a structured training programme. While it is moderately sensitive for detecting solid organ injury, FAST scanning rarely detects injury to a hollow viscus even in experienced hands.

1.   Salomone   JA.   Blunt   abdominal   trauma.   Available: http://www.emedicine.com/emerg/topic1.htm. Last accessed 20 November 2008.

K55   TTFT

The diaphragm extends from the 4th intercostal space anteriorly to the 7th posteriorly. A stab wound could easily cause tension pneumothorax or cardiac tamponade, both of which should be excluded clinically, then radiologically. There may be more stab wounds or other injuries which should be identified prior to laparotomy as they may be occult sources of blood loss. Although a positive FAST scan has a high positive predictive value for therapeutic laparotomy, a negative scan does not negate the need for laparotomy in the presence of clinical signs of intraperitoneal injury. Haemodynamic instability or peritonism are absolute indications for laparotomy in penetrating abdominal injury. While 'hypotensive resuscitation' has a place in penetrating trauma, fluid should be titrated to achieve an adequate blood pressure (often taken as 90mmHg systolic) or clear consciousness. There is no indication to omit fluids in this shocked patient.

1.   Testa PA. Abdominal trauma, penetrating. Available: http://www.emedicine.com/emerg/topic2.htm. Last accessed 20 November 2008.

K56   TTTF

Abdominal compartment syndrome (ACS) can be primary (due to an intra-abdominal cause, e.g. pancreatitis, haemorrhage, trauma, perforation), or secondary to high-volume fluid resuscitation, extensive burns or sepsis (any condition where capillary leak can cause large volumes of fluid to be sequestered in the abdominal compartment). Laparostomy is the treatment for ACS, but is not without complications including infection, extensive fluid losses, evisceration, bleeding, postoperative hernias and small bowel obstruction.

1.   Bailey J, Shapiro MJ. Abdominal compartment syndrome. *Crit Care* 2000; 4: 23-9.

K57   TTTT

The normal range varies between institutions, but is around 0.2-0.4g/L. Elevated CSF protein is extremely non-specific and may signify any of the causes above, as well as abscess, haemorrhage, demyelinating disease and Guillain-Barré syndrome. Causes of low CSF protein include a chronic dural leak or repeated lumbar punctures, and water intoxication. Hypoproteinaemia is not a cause, however.

1. Seehusen DA, Reeves MM, Fomin DA. Cerebrospinal fluid analysis. *Am Fam Physician* 2003; 68(6): 1103-8.

K58   TFTF

This history is highly suggestive of the serotonin syndrome. This is a dose-related hypermetabolic condition characterised by mental state changes, autonomic hyperactivity and neuromuscular changes, although not all three are always present. Both selective serotonin reuptake inhibitor (SSRI) antidepressants and ecstasy could cause such a presentation. Benzodiazepines may be used to control agitation, but in severe cases with muscular rigidity and high pyrexia, intubation, mechanical ventilation and full supportive care are required. A 5-HT2A antagonist, cyproheptadine, is also a recommended treatment.

1. Boyer EW, Shannon M. The serotonin syndrome. *New Engl J Med* 2005; 352: 1112-20.

K59   FFFT

The history suggests toxic megacolon on a background of pseudomembranous colitis secondary to recent treatment with broad spectrum antibiotics. This is a surgical emergency and may complicate any form of colitis including inflammatory bowel disease and ischaemia. If treatment with oral metronidazole and/or vancomycin does not produce swift improvement, colectomy or a defunctioning ileostomy may be needed. Clindamycin, amoxycillin and cephalosporins are common causes of pseudomembranous colitis. Mortality is currently around 5% (this figure has fallen with better ICU management and prompt surgical intervention).

1.   Sheth SG. LaMont JT. Toxic megacolon. *Lancet* 1998; 351: 509-12.

K60   FTFF

Evidence for a mortality benefit from recombinant human activated protein C (rhAPC) comes from two randomised controlled trials. The PROWESS trial enrolled 1690 patients with sepsis and organ failure who were randomised to receive a 96-hour infusion of either rhAPC (24µg/kg/h) or placebo. The 28-day all-cause mortality was reduced from 30.8% to 24.7% (a relative risk reduction of 19.4%). Subgroup analysis suggested that patients with a higher risk of death (measured by higher APACHE II scores or greater number organ failures) gained the greatest benefit. The subsequent ADDRESS trial enrolled 2613 patients with sepsis and a low risk of death (APACHE II score <25 or single organ failure) and showed no mortality benefit with rhAPC. The drug is currently licensed for patients with a high risk of death (APACHE II scores >25 or multiple organ failure). A variety of other 'magic bullets' for sepsis have been trialled with disappointing results, including antithrombin III, heparin, anti-tumour necrosis factor antibodies and interleukin-1 receptor antagonists.

1.   Bersten AD, Soni N. *Oh's Intensive Care Manual*, 5th Ed. Edinburgh: Butterworth-Heinemann, 2003.
2.   Bernard GR, *et al.* Efficacy and safety of recombinant human activated protein C for severe sepsis. *N Engl J Med* 2001; 344(10): 699-709.
3.   Abraham E, *et al.* Drotrecogin alfa (activated) for adults with severe sepsis and a low risk of death. *N Engl J Med* 2005; 353(13): 1332-41.

K61   FFTT

This man has a coagulopathy as indicated by the bleeding, raised INR and low platelet count. While recombinant factor VIIa is an option in major blunt trauma, correction of platelets, fibrinogen, hypothermia, acidosis and ionised calcium to minimum levels is a pre-requisite for its use. Vitamin K will be of little benefit since the problem is a dilutional coagulopathy in a man who has received a massive transfusion of (clotting factor-deficient) packed red cells, rather than a primary synthetic problem. He is likely to be hypothermic which will exacerbate his coagulopathy, and strenuous efforts should be made to re-warm him. Under the ATLS® classification of shock, class III implies blood loss of 1500-2000ml.

1. Spahn DR, *et al*. Management of bleeding following major trauma: a European guideline. *Crit Care* 2007; 11(1): R17.

K62   TTFT

Patients with a coagulopathy in the context of major trauma have a worse outcome than those with the same injury severity without a clotting disturbance. An isolated haematocrit is not a sensitive indicator of the presence of traumatic haemorrhage; while patients with major haemorrhage may have serially reducing haematocrit measurements, a patient with serious bleeding may maintain their haematocrit level, especially if blood products have been transfused. Venous and cancellous bone bleeding following pelvic fracture may be devastating, and is reduced by pelvic fixation, either surgically with an external fixation device, or by the use of a bed sheet or pelvic binder. A shocked patient will have a reduced cardiac output. Venous return to the heart will be further compromised by high levels of PEEP, which should be minimised until bleeding has been controlled.

1. Spahn DR, *et al*. Management of bleeding following major trauma: a European guideline. *Crit Care* 2007; 11(1): R17.

K63   FFFF

Clinical estimation of the body surface area (BSA) of a burn injury is notoriously unreliable. It may be estimated using a Lund and Browder chart or simplified 'rule of nines' chart (see Figure overleaf). From the description given in the question, this man has approximately 36% BSA burns. 4mL/kg/% burned BSA of crystalloid given over 24 hours would be

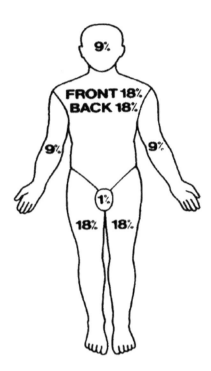

a reasonable fluid strategy from the time of the burn injury, not from arrival in hospital. Suxamethonium can cause life-threatening hyperkalaemia from about 10 days post-burn by stimulation of extra-junctional acetylcholine receptors which develop. It is safe at the time of the injury. This patient has signs of smoke inhalation and probably has significant carbon monoxide poisoning. Arterial PaO_2 may not reflect blood oxygen carriage, and 100% O_2 is warranted initially to reduce carboxyhaemoglobin levels.

1. Mackie DP. Burns. In: *Oh's Intensive Care Manual*, 5th Ed. Bersten AD, Soni N, Eds. Edinburgh: Butterworth-Heinemann, 2003.

K64 FFTF

ESBL production confers resistance against all third generation cephalosporins including cefotaxime, ceftriaxone and ceftazidime. Fourth generation cephalosporins (cefepime) are much less susceptible to ESBL *in vitro*, but may not be as effective *in vivo* and should not be used as first-line treatment. Although ESBL producers are susceptible to ß-lactam/ß-lactamase inhibitor combinations *in vitro*, the ß-lactamase inhibitor may be overwhelmed by the concentration of ESBL *in vivo*, and therefore clinical effect is much less impressive; combination with an aminoglycoside is recommended. Although ESBL has no effect on aminoglycosides, the plasmid which codes for this commonly confers resistance to this class of antibiotic also (16.1 % of ESBL-producers were resistant to gentamicin in one study); they should not be used as monotherapy. Fluoroquinolone resistance is equally common. Carbapenems have good *in vitro* and *in vivo* effect against ESBL producers and are the antibiotics of first choice if serious infection with an ESBL-producing organism is suspected.

1.   Sturenburg E, Mack D. Extended-spectrum ß-lactamases: implications for the clinical microbiology laboratory, therapy, and infection control. *Journal of Infection* 2003; 47: 273-95.

K65   FTTF

The FTc is low, reflecting increased systemic vascular resistance (SVR). The clinical history suggests this is due to cardiac failure (not all cases of reduced FTc are due to hypovolaemia [1]). There is a lack of response to a fluid challenge (no significant increase in stroke volume, decrease in peak velocity) suggesting that this patient is fluid-overloaded and 'over the top' of the Starling curve. Nitrates and frusemide would be appropriate therapy to offload the left ventricle. Peak velocity gives some indication of cardiac contractility. The normal range for a patient of this age is 50-70cm/s. If this does not improve with offloading measures, inotropic support may be indicated.

1.   Singer M. The FTc is not an accurate marker of left ventricular preload. *Intensive Care Med* 2006; 32: 1089.

K66   TFFT

Pulse pressure is directly proportional to stroke volume, and inversely related to the compliance of the arterial tree. Changes in pulse pressure across the respiratory cycle therefore reflect changes in stroke volume. A change in pulse pressure (ΔPP) >13% in a mechanically ventilated patient is a sensitive and specific indicator of a positive response to a fluid challenge. Systolic pressure variation (ΔSP) is less useful, since part of the variation is due to factors other than stroke volume changes such as the cyclic direct effects of intrathoracic pressure on the thoracic aorta wall. At peak inspiratory pressure, there is a brief increase in systolic pressure (Δup) caused in part by transiently increased left ventricular preload as blood is squeezed out of the pulmonary veins. The fall in systolic pressure (Δdown) comes a few heartbeats later as the effects of reduced right heart preload are transmitted to the left heart; this coincides temporally with expiration. ΔPP and ΔSP are unreliable in arrhythmias such as atrial fibrillation.

1.   Lamia B, *et al.* Clinical review: interpretation of arterial pressure wave in shock states. *Crit Care* 2005; 9: 601-6.

K67   FTTF

The resonant (or natural) frequency of a measuring system is that frequency at which the undamped transducer system oscillates with maximal amplitude. If the resonant frequency is within the clinical range of input frequencies, excessive oscillation (resonance) will occur, with overestimation of systolic and underestimation of diastolic pressures. The resonant frequency should be at least 10 times the fundamental frequency (or primary harmonic). This is the lowest frequency that can be used to describe the arterial pressure trace. For arterial blood pressure measurement the normal range is 60-120 beats per minute (i.e. the primary harmonic is 1-2Hz). The connecting tubing should be short, stiff and wide to ensure that the resonant frequency is above the clinically encountered range. Damping is the process whereby some of the energy of the oscillations produced within the measuring system is absorbed, thus reducing their amplitude. A certain amount of damping is desirable to minimise excessive oscillation. Bubbles, clots and kinks may cause excessive damping of the signal however.

1.   Stoker MR. Principles of pressure transducers, resonance, damping and frequency response. *Anaesthesia and Intensive Care* 2004; 5(11): 371-5.

K68 FFTT

The Richmond agitation and sedation scale is scored from +4 (combative and violent) to -5 (unrousable). A score of 0 (alert and calm) is desirable. Although ICU delirium may present as hyperarousal and agitation, a withdrawn, hypoactive form is much more common albeit under-recognised. The Ramsay sedation scale is the most frequently used sedation scoring system in clinical investigations, but does not assess agitation. It is primarily a test of rousability. A score from 1 (anxious and restless) to 6 (unresponsive) is given, with 3-4 being optimal. The GCS is a test of neurological function and is not useful in the assessment of sedation.

1.   Cullis B, Macnaughton P. Sedation and neuromuscular paralysis in the ICU. *Anaesthesia & Intensive Care Medicine* 2006; 8(1): 32-5.

K69 FTTT

Excessive heparinisation of a blood sample allows the blood to equilibrate with a volume of fluid which has a very low partial pressure of CO_2 and a PaO_2 of around 21kPa, assuming the heparin has itself equilibrated with room air. Therefore, measured $PaCO_2$ will always be lowered, and measured PaO_2 may be falsely low or high, depending on the true PaO_2 of the blood with which it is equilibrated. Although heparin is acidic, the buffering power of haemoglobin and plasma proteins is such that the effect on pH is negligible. Since bicarbonate is calculated by the blood gas analyser from the Henderson-Hasselbach equation, a fall in measured $PaCO_2$ will cause a proportionate fall in calculated bicarbonate.

1.   Dake MD, Peters J, Teague R. The effect of heparin dilution on arterial blood gas analysis. *West J Med* 1984; 140(5): 792-4.

K70 FFTF

While mild hypothermia may be treated with passive re-warming, active methods should be employed for moderate and severe hypothermia. This man has a reduced GCS, bradycardia and a low temperature and is in the latter category. Intubation should be performed if indicated since the risk of precipitating VF with necessary procedures is actually small. In thiamine-deficient patients (malnourished/alcoholic patients), re-warming may precipitate Wernicke's encephalopathy and thiamine should be given immediately. Cardioversion can be attempted below 30°C, but if a perfusing rhythm is not restored after three shocks no further attempts should be made until core temperature is above 30°C.

1.   Epstein E, Anna A. Accidental hypothermia. *BMJ* 2006; 332: 706-9.

K71   FFTT

Focal cognitive impairment is in keeping with delirium, whereas global impairment suggests dementia. The onset of symptoms is typically acute with delirium (hours), but insidious with dementia. Inattention is a cardinal feature of delirium and must be actively sought (e.g. unable to recite a short series of numbers backwards). Psychotic symptoms may be part of dementia, but are far more common in delirium. It is worth noting that many patients have an acute delirium superimposed upon a chronic dementing process. Dementia predisposes to delirium in the critically ill patient (five-fold increased risk); 30-40% of delirious patients have underlying dementia.

1.   Borthwick M, *et al.* Detection, prevention and treatment of delirium in critically ill patients. United Kingdom Clinical Pharmacy Association, 2006. [Available from the Intensive Care Society website at: www.ics.ac.uk].
2.   Inouye SK. A practical program for preventing delirium in hospitalized elderly patients. *Cleveland Clinic Journal of Medicine* 2004; 71(11): 890-6.

K72   TFTF

In the past acute epiglottitis was largely a disease of children, but with the advent of routine childhood immunization against *H. influenzae* B, adults are now more commonly affected with a male: female ratio of 2.5:1. Common pathogens are *H. influenzae* (25% of cases), *H. parainfluenzae*, *Streptococcus pneumoniae* and *Streptococcus pyogenes*. In many cases no pathogen is identified. Sore throat, dysphagia and odynophagia (pain on swallowing) are almost always present, and patients are usually toxic and unwell with a high fever. A prodromal upper respiratory tract illness may be present. Death occurring from airway obstruction has been reported even in patients monitored closely on the ICU, and a low threshold for securing a definitive airway should be present. Amoxycillin with clavulanic acid or a third generation cephalosporin are appropriate empirical treatments.

1. Sack JL, Brock CD. Identifying acute epiglottitis in adults. *Postgrad Med* 2002; 112(1): 81-2.

K73 TFTT

There are several contraindications to thrombolysis, of which intracranial bleeding is probably the strongest. In such cases, where further pulmonary embolism might be lethal, placement of a vena cava filter may be appropriate. Such filters may be permanent, but some are removable and have been removed up to a year after placement. Although vena cava filters reduce further pulmonary emboli, they increase the risk of deep vein thrombosis and have not been demonstrated to improve survival.

1. Tapson VF. Acute pulmonary embolism. *New Engl J Med* 2008; 358(10): 1037-52.

K74 FTTT

Hyperventilation to a $PaCO_2$ of below 4.0kPa (30mmHg) is not recommended for the routine management of head injury patients, since it causes cerebral artery vasoconstriction and may worsen brain ischaemia. However, as an acute measure it will reduce intracranial pressure and may buy time until definitive treatment. Mannitol is the most commonly used diuretic, with other effects including removal of fluid from the brain via osmotic shift (assuming an intact blood-brain barrier) and free radical scavenging. Frusemide is also acceptable, however. Although thiopentone is not usually used for routine sedation due to its long and unpredictable half-life, a thiopentone coma will reduce cerebral blood volume and, hence, intracranial pressure by flow-metabolism coupling. There is no place for dobutamine in the management of raised intracranial pressure.

1. Dunn LT. Raised intracranial pressure. *J Neurol Neurosurg Psychiatry* 2002; 73: 23-7.

K75 FTTF

A rapid fall in the end-tidal CO_2 over the course of a few breaths indicates a fall in cardiac output causing a large increase in physiological dead space (increased V/Q ratio). This can be caused by a large air embolism or pulmonary embolism, or a fall in cardiac output due to any cause (cardiogenic shock, hypovolaemia, anaphylaxis, etc). Endobronchial intubation would not affect the capnography trace initially, although with time the end-tidal CO_2 would rise due to the reduced minute volume. Bronchospasm would alter the shape of the waveform characteristically (rising to a peak rather than being 'flat-topped').

1. Hutton P. Monitoring and safety. In: *Fundamental Principles and Practice of Anaesthesia*. Hutton P, Cooper GM, James FM, Butterworth JF, Eds. London: Taylor-Francis, 2002.

K76 FTFF

This lady has a history supporting a diagnosis of ventricular septal rupture as a consequence of recent anterior myocardial infarction (MI). Septal rupture results in a left-to-right shunt with right ventricular volume overload, increased pulmonary blood flow and secondary left heart volume overload. It usually occurs within a week of MI, sooner if thrombolysis has been given, and a harsh systolic murmur is characteristic. Doppler echocardiography is diagnostic, and excludes papillary muscle rupture, a major differential diagnosis. ECG is not diagnostic, but may show atrioventricular block in a third of patients. Pulmonary artery catheter data show a step increase in right ventricular and pulmonary artery oxygen saturation due to the shunt (higher than right atrial saturation), and raised pulmonary artery pressures. In this case the pulmonary artery SpO_2 of 88% is much higher than would normally be expected (mixed venous oxygen saturation should be around 70%), strongly suggesting the presence of a left-to-right shunt and not explained by papillary muscle rupture. Medical management includes afterload reduction (to reduce the shunt), diuretics and an intra-aortic balloon pump. Surgical repair is usually required; the 30-day survival rate is only 24% with medical management and 47% when treated surgically. Systemic hypotension and high right atrial pressure confers a grave prognosis. Needle thoracocentesis would be the treatment of choice for cardiac tamponade; while this may cause distended neck veins, the presence of a loud murmur and the pulmonary artery catheter data do not support this diagnosis.

1. Birnbaum Y, *et al.* Ventricular septal rupture after acute myocardial infarction. *New Engl J Med* 2002; 347: 1426-32.

K77   FFTT

Death in such cases is usually from asphyxiation rather than exsanguination. The first priority is to secure the airway and improve this patient's oxygenation. Initially it may be better to use a standard endotracheal tube as this will allow rapid airway control and facilitate passage of the bronchoscope for diagnostic and therapeutic manoeuvres. The patient should be ventilated with the bleeding side dependent if this is known, to prevent blood from contaminating the other lung. Fibreoptic bronchoscopy may be difficult or impossible due to blood obscuring the field of view, but should be attempted by an experienced operator. It may be possible to perform bronchial toilet, identify a source of bleeding and conduct therapeutic manoeuvres such as intrabronchial iced saline lavage or topical epinephrine infusion. While a double-lumen tube has the obvious advantage of isolating the bleeding lung, it has lumens of narrow diameter which may become occluded with clots. Moreover, therapeutic deployment of the fibreoptic bronchoscope through a double-lumen tube may be difficult or impossible. The best course of action may be to use a standard endotracheal tube initially and then replace it with a double-lumen tube once control has been gained and the bronchoscope deployed.

1. Hakanson E, *et al.* Management of life-threatening haemoptysis. *Br J Anaesth* 2002; 88(2): 291-5.

K78   FFTF

The only ventilatory strategy proven to significantly reduce mortality in ARDS is the use of low tidal volumes and limiting plateau pressure. A large multicentre ARDSNet trial [1] demonstrated an absolute reduction in hospital mortality rate of 9% (31% vs 39.8%) in patients ventilated with a tidal volume of ≤6ml/kg predicted body weight and a plateau pressure of ≤30cmH$_2$O compared with controls ventilated with tidal volumes of 12ml/kg. None of the other manoeuvres in the question have a proven mortality benefit, although all improve short-term oxygenation and are frequently used as rescue therapy.

1. The Acute Respiratory Distress Syndrome Network. Ventilation with lower tidal volumes as compared with traditional tidal volumes for acute lung injury and the acute respiratory distress syndrome. *N Engl J Med* 2000; 342: 1301-8.
2. Girard TD, Bernard GR. Mechanical ventilation in ARDS: a state-of-the-art review. *Chest* 2007; 131: 921-9.

K79   TTTF

Postoperative atrial fibrillation most commonly occurs on the first postoperative day. It is very common following cardiac surgery (25-40%) and thoracic surgery (40%), but much lower in non-cardiac, non-thoracic surgery (0.4% overall, higher in major abdominal and vascular procedures). The risk of stroke is increased three-fold, and the risk of other postoperative complications such as myocardial infarction and congestive cardiac failure also increases. It resolves spontaneously in most patients, however. Risk factors include older age, valvular heart disease, atrial enlargement and chronic lung disease.

1. Cavaliere F, *et al*. Atrial fibrillation in intensive care units. *Current Anaesthesia & Critical Care* 2006; 17: 367-74.

K80   TTFF

Acute coronary syndrome (ACS) is a clinical diagnosis made on the basis of history and ECG findings. Elevated cardiac enzymes may indicate a non-ST-segment elevation myocardial infarction (one end of the spectrum of ACS). The key to management of ACS is risk stratification. Older age (>65 years), new ST depression, pre-existing angina and prolonged chest pain (>20 minutes) are all associated with increased cardiac risk. Various scoring systems are available to risk-stratify patients based on these and other factors. Low-risk patients should be treated non-invasively and may be risk-stratified further with early exercise stress testing. High-risk patients should undergo early (inpatient) angiography to assess suitability for revascularisation and should be started on glycoprotein IIb/IIIa inhibitors. These drugs (e.g. eptifibatide, tirofiban) reduce the 30-day risk of death or non-fatal myocardial infarction by 1%, but increase the incidence of major bleeding by 1%. In high-risk groups, however, the benefits are greater. In general, aspirin should be administered to all patients with suspected ACS. Clopidogrel has been shown to confer an additional benefit over aspirin alone [1], and should be administered to patients with ACS and no contraindications. All patients should also receive either low-molecular-weight or unfractionated heparin.

1. Fox KAA, et al. Benefits and risks of the combination of clopidogrel and aspirin in patients undergoing surgical revascularization for non-ST-elevation acute coronary syndrome. The Clopidogrel in Unstable angina to prevent Recurrent ischemic Events (CURE) Trial. *Circulation* 2004; 110: 1202-8.
2. Anderson JL, et al. ACC/AHA 2007 guidelines for the management of patients with unstable angina/non-ST-elevation myocardial infarction. *J Am Coll Cardiol* 2007; 50: 1-157.

K81 TFTT

The commonest cause of cardiogenic shock is anterior myocardial infarction. Left ventricular 'pump failure' is responsible for the majority of cases of cardiogenic shock (about 80%), but other causes include mitral regurgitation, cardiac tamponade and right ventricular failure. Both mechanical ventilation and CPAP increase intrathoracic pressure. This reduces venous return and therefore preload, which is usually beneficial in cardiogenic shock. In addition, afterload is reduced, since this is determined by the transmural pressure across the wall of the left ventricle, which falls with the increase in intrathoracic pressure. Both these factors will tend to increase cardiac output; in addition, the work of breathing is greatly reduced, reducing the blood flow requirements of the diaphragm and respiratory muscles.

1. Boehmer JP, Popjes E. Cardiac failure: mechanical support strategies. *Crit Care Med* 2006; 34(9): S268-78.

K82   TTFF

Cavernous sinus thrombosis is rare, accounting for around 3% of cases of cerebral venous sinus thrombosis. It is characterised by painful ophthalmoplegia, proptosis and chemosis. The location of the cavernous sinuses and their extensive venous connections makes them vulnerable to septic thrombi from infection at multiple sites. This may be local (e.g. sinusitis of the ethmoid or sphenoid sinuses) or distant. The commonest pathogen is *Staphylococcus aureus*, found in 60-70% of cases. In the pre-antibiotic era, mortality was 80-100%, but this has fallen to ~20% with appropriate antimicrobial therapy. Long-term sequalae are not uncommon in survivors, however. A high resolution CT brain scan is a useful investigation, and may show enlargement or expansion of the cavernous sinuses with filling defects on contrast injection. Magnetic resonance scanning may occasionally be required if CT fails to make the diagnosis.

1.   Ebright JR, *et al.* Septic thrombosis of the cavernous sinuses. *Arch Intern Med* 2001; 161: 2671-6.

K83   TTTT

Weakness following critical illness is common and multifactorial. Estimates of incidence vary between 33-82% in patients ventilated for >4-7 days. Nerve conduction studies frequently show evidence of denervation, while muscle biopsy shows evidence of myopathy. It may be that neuromuscular function is yet another manifestation of the multiple organ failure associated with the systemic inflammatory response. The factors listed in the question are the major associations with weakness following intensive care. The only intervention that has been shown to reduce the incidence of critical illness polyneuromyopathy is tight glycaemic control. In a study of surgical ICU patients [1], maintenance of serum glucose between 4.4-6mmol/L (80-110mg/dL) reduced electrophysiologically diagnosed polyneuropathy by 49%.

1.   Van den Berghe G, Wouters P, Weekers F, Verwaest C, Bruyninckx F, Schetz M, *et al.* Intensive insulin therapy in the critically ill patients. *N Engl J Med* 2001; 345(19): 1359-67.

2.   Deem S. Intensive care unit-acquired muscle weakness. *Resp Care* 2006; 51(9): 1042-53.

K84   TFFF

Red cell casts are formed from glomerular bleeding, and not from other sources of bleeding in the urogenital tract. This may reflect glomerulonephritis or nephritic syndrome. Nitrite is formed from the bacterial reduction of urinary nitrates. Although 90% of common urinary pathogens are nitrite-forming, *Pseudomonas spp.*, *Staphylococcus albus*, *Staphylococcus saprophyticus*, and *Streptococcus faecalis* may have minimal or no nitrite-producing capacity. Nitrite dipstick testing has been shown to be an insensitive indicator of the presence of bacteriuria. Hyaline casts are composed of Tamm-Horsfall glycoprotein, secreted by the cells of the distal nephron. This is a common finding in healthy individuals. In some cases of bacterial endocarditis, red cell casts may be present due to associated glomerulonephritis. White cell casts are found in proliferative glomerulonephritis, acute interstitial nephritis and acute pyelonephritis.

1. Davenport A. Clinical investigation of renal disease. In: *Oxford Textbook of Medicine*. Warrell D, Cox TM, Firth JD, Benz EJ, Eds. Oxford: Oxford University Press [Online Edition], 2004.

K85   FFTF

Sucralfate forms a protective barrier over the surface of the stomach reducing exposure to acidic gastric contents. It has no effect on gastric pH, however. When compared with H_2-receptor antagonists, proton pump inhibitors seem to be more effective in reducing gastric acidity, but have not been demonstrated to be superior preventing clinically significant bleeding. Tolerance occurs to ranitidine but not to proton pump inhibitors. Antacids have some effect in reducing stress ulceration provided gastric pH is kept above 3.5, but frequent dosing (2-hourly) is required to achieve this goal, making their use impractical.

1. Stollman N, Metz DC. Pathophysiology and prophylaxis of stress ulcer in intensive care unit patients. *Journal of Critical Care* 2005; 20: 35-45.

K86 TFTF

Acute intestinal pseudo-obstruction (Ogilvie's syndrome [1]) is characterised by impairment of intestinal propulsion in the absence of a mechanical cause. It may present following a medical or surgical insult such as myocardial infarction, stroke, major surgery, sepsis or trauma. Discomfort is usual, but severe pain is more suggestive of perforation or ischaemia. Dilated large bowel loops with air in the rectosigmoid colon on plain abdominal radiography confirm the diagnosis, but the absence of air does not differentiate between pseudo-obstruction and mechanical obstruction. Free passage of contrast on enema studies differentiates between the two conditions with high sensitivity and specificity. Colonic diameter correlates with the likelihood of perforation, and surgical intervention should be considered if >9cm. It does not differentiate between the two pathologies, however. Bowel sounds may be present or absent with pseudo-obstruction.

1. Ogilvie H. Large intestine colic due to sympathetic deprivation: a new clinical syndrome. *BMJ* 1948; 2: 671-3.
2. Delgado-Aros S, Camilleri M. Pseudo-obstruction in the critically ill. *Best Prac Res Clin Gastroent* 2003; 17(3): 427-44.

K87 TTTT

Uraemic gastroparesis can alter the absorption of various drugs such as short-acting sulphonylureas. Vomiting and diarrhoea are also common and can reduce the absorption of drugs from the gastrointestinal tract. Hypoalbuminaemia can affect the protein binding of acidic drugs, increasing the free fraction of drugs such as phenytoin. Tissue oedema due to excess total body water may increase the volume of distribution (Vd) of water-soluble drugs such as vancomycin, which will require a greater loading dose to achieve therapeutic levels. Tissue protein binding is reduced in uraemic states, reducing the Vd of highly-tissue protein-bound drugs such as digoxin. Renal failure can influence the hepatic metabolism of drugs by effects on the cytochrome p450 enzyme family. Some drugs have increased hepatic metabolism (e.g. nifedipine), whereas others exhibit reduced hepatic metabolism (e.g. metoclopramide, nicardipine). Glomerular filtration and tubular secretion are reduced in renal failure decreasing elimination of many drugs.

1. Elston AC, Bayliss MK, Park GR. Effect of renal failure on drug metabolism by the liver. Br J Anaesth 1993; 71: 282-90.
2. Kappel J, Calissi P. Nephrology: 3. Safe drug prescribing for patients with renal insufficiency. CMAJ 2002; 166(4): 473-7.

K88   TFTF

Propranolol is the mainstay of prophylaxis against bleeding for gastro-oesophageal varices. It causes splanchnic vasoconstriction, lowering variceal pressure. Meta-analysis of several randomised trials has shown that propranolol reduces the risk of significant bleeding, and may confer a mortality benefit. It is not indicated for the emergency treatment of active variceal bleeding, however. Patients who are intolerant of beta-blockade may benefit from slow-release nitrates which lower portal venous pressure. Again, this is useful as prophylaxis rather than treatment of an acute bleed. Glypressin is a synthetic vasopressin analogue which reduces portal blood flow and variceal pressure. It has been shown to improve survival and be as effective as balloon tamponade for bleeding control. Somatostatin causes selective splanchnic vasoconstriction and reduces portal pressure. It compares favourably with balloon tamponade and vasopressin, and causes less cardiovascular disturbance than the latter.

1. Jalan R, Hayes PC. UK guidelines on the management of variceal haemorrhage in cirrhotic patients. Gut 2000; 46: 1-15.

K89   FFTT

Numerous meta-analyses have compared total parenteral nutrition (TPN) with enteral nutrition. Recent evidence suggests that overall, TPN is associated with a lower mortality rate than enteral feeding [1]. This effect is only observed when TPN is compared with delayed enteral feeding, however; when early enteral and parenteral feeding are compared, no mortality difference is seen [1, 2]. The rate of infectious complications and length of hospital stay are significantly greater with TPN; this may reflect the fact that TPN is often instituted in sicker patients. When comparing early enteral nutrition with delayed enteral nutrition, infectious complications and hospital length of stay are reduced, but no mortality benefit is seen [3]. The consensus view is that early enteral nutrition should be instituted if possible, with TPN being commenced if enteral feeding has not been established within 24 hours of admission.

1. Simpson F, Doig GS. Parenteral vs. enteral nutrition in the critically ill patient: a meta-analysis of trials using the intention to treat principle. *Intensive Care Med* 2005; 31(1): 12-23.
2. Peter JV, *et al.* A meta-analysis of treatment outcomes of early enteral versus early parenteral nutrition in hospitalized patients. *Crit Care Med* 2005; 33(1): 213-20.
3. Marik PE, Zaloga GP. Early enteral nutrition in acutely ill patients: a systematic review. *Crit Care Med* 2001; 29(12): 2264-70.

K90   TFFT

The 24-hour sepsis management bundle is a package of evidence-based measures designed to reduce mortality in patients with septic shock as advocated by the Surviving Sepsis Campaign (SSC). This bundle is distilled from the wider recommendations of the SSC as an achievable package that can be put in place for all septic patients. Activated protein C should be considered for all patients meeting the specified criteria. Low-dose corticosteroids should be administered to patients with shock requiring vasopressor support (hydrocortisone 200-300mg/day). Glucose should be maintained between 3.8-8.3mmol/L (70-150mg/dL). Plateau pressure should be maintained below 30cmH$_2$O for mechanically ventilated patients.

1. Dellinger RP, *et al* for the International Surviving Sepsis Campaign Guidelines Committee. Surviving Sepsis Campaign: International guidelines for management of severe sepsis and septic shock: 2008. *Crit Care Med* 2008; 36(1): 296-327.

K91   TTFT

The Sequential Organ Failure Assessment (SOFA) score [1] was developed to assess and track organ dysfunction over time. The SOFA score quantifies morbidity, but does not predict outcome, although a clear relationship between SOFA score and mortality has been demonstrated in several studies [2].

Table 1. SOFA score.

Organ system	Parameter	SOFA score				
		0	1	2	3	4
Respiratory	PaO₂:FiO₂ ratio,	>400	<400	<300	<200	<100
	mmHg (kPa)	(>53)	(<53)	(<39.5)	(<26.3)	(<13.2)
Coagulation	Platelets x 10³/μL	>150	<150	<100	<50	<20
Liver	Bilirubin μmol/L	<20	20-33	34-100	101-203	>12
	(mg/dL)	(<1.2)	(1.2-1.9)	(2.0-5.9)	(6.0-11.9)	(>203)
Cardiovascular	Blood pressure, vasoactive drugs	No hypo -tension	MAP<70 mmHg	Increasing levels of inotropic /vasopressor support		
CNS	Glasgow Coma Score	15	14-13	12-10	9-6	<6
Renal	Creatinine μmol/L	<106	106-168	168-301	301-433	>433
	(mg/dL)	(<1.2)	(1.2-1.9)	(2.0-3.4)	(3.5-4.9)	(>5.0)

1. Vincent JL, Moreno R, Takala J, *et al*, for the Working Group on Sepsis-Related Problems of the European Society of Intensive Care Medicine. The SOFA (Sepsis-related Organ Failure Assessment) score to describe organ dysfunction/failure. *Intensive Care Med* 1996; 22: 707-10.
2. Ferreira FL, *et al*. Serial evaluation of the SOFA score to predict outcome in critically ill patients. *JAMA* 2001; 286(14): 1754-8.

K92 TFFT

HFOV delivers extremely high frequency (>3-15Hz) low tidal volume (<3ml/kg) breaths. A pressurised circuit is generated by a continuous flow of gas (bias flow) and a control valve. An electronically-controlled diaphragm vibrates in and out at high speed causing oscillations in circuit pressure (ΔP) around the mean airway pressure. Although ΔP may be very high (>60cmH$_2$O) when measured in the breathing circuit, this pressure is significantly attenuated by various factors including the diameter of the endotracheal tube, the compliance of the respiratory system, airway resistance and the frequency of oscillation. Increasing the mean airway pressure improves oxygenation by greater splinting open of alveoli (with reduced shunt). Expiration is active (the diaphragm moves both 'in' and 'out'). A typical frequency of ventilation is 5Hz (300 breaths/min). Elimination of CO_2 can be increased by either increasing ΔP or decreasing the frequency, both of which will increase the degree of ΔP transmitted to the small airways and increase the tidal volume.

1. Pillow JJ. High-frequency oscillatory ventilator ventilation: mechanisms of gas exchange and lung mechanics. *Crit Care Med* 2005; 33(3): S135-41.
2. Krishnan JA, Brower RG. High-frequency ventilation for acute lung injury and ARDS. *Chest* 2000; 118: 795-807.

K93 TTTT

Obstructive shock and cardiogenic shock are thought to predominate early in the course of an amniotic fluid embolism. The former appears due to intense pulmonary artery vasoconstriction on exposure to immunologically active substances. Left ventricular dysfunction is frequently seen on echocardiography. Later in the course of the syndrome a distributive shock state supervenes as part of a generalised systemic inflammatory response with capillary leak. Disseminated intravascular coagulation is a common complication of amniotic fluid embolism (present in >80% of patients), and life-threatening haemorrhage may occur.

1. Moore J, Baldisseri MR. Amniotic fluid embolism. *Crit Care Med* 2005; 33(10): S279-85.

K94 TTTF

Several large randomised controlled trials (including the VIGOR [1] and TARGET [2] trials) have shown that COX-2 inhibitors reduce the risk of gastrointestinal complications, including ulceration and bleeding by around half compared with non-selective non-steroidal anti-inflammatory drugs (NSAIDs). Several large trials have shown an increased risk of cardiovascular adverse events (myocardial infarction and stroke) with COX-2 inhibitors compared with non-selective NSAIDs. One possible explanation for this is that COX-2 inhibition reduces prostacyclin production in vascular endothelium (which has vasodilatory and antiplatelet activity) and increases thromboxane A_2 production (pro-aggregatory platelet effects). Rofecoxib was shown to increase the risk of myocardial infarction by a factor of 2.3 in a recent meta-analysis [3] and appears to be more strongly associated with problems than other agents in the same class. The evidence in this area is complicated, however, and it may be the case that even non-selective NSAIDs increase the cardiovascular risk to some degree. COX-2 inhibitors are contraindicated in the UK for patients with a history of ischaemic heart disease, cerebrovascular disease or active heart failure. They may be suitable for those with musculoskeletal pain who are susceptible to gastrointestinal side effects with traditional NSAIDs. The analgesic efficacy of COX-2 agents is among the highest of all NSAIDs.

1. Bombardier C, *et al*; VIGOR Study Group. Comparison of upper gastrointestinal toxicity of rofecoxib and naproxen in patients with rheumatoid arthritis. VIGOR Study Group. *N Engl J Med* 2000; 343: 1520-8.
2. Schnitzer TJ, *et al*; TARGET Study Group. Comparison of lumiracoxib with naproxen and ibuprofen in the Therapeutic Arthritis Research and Gastrointestinal Event Trial (TARGET), reduction in ulcer complications: randomised controlled trial. *Lancet* 2004; 364: 665-74.
3. Juni P, *et al*. Risk of cardiovascular events and rofecoxib: cumulative meta-analysis. *Lancet* 2004; 364: 2021-9.
4. Ong CKS, *et al*. An evidence-based update on nonsteroidal anti-inflammatory drugs. *Clin Med Res* 2007; 5(1): 19-34.

K95   FTFT

The half-life of a drug is the time taken for its concentration to fall by 50%. The initial volume of distribution is as stated following a bolus dose of an intravenous drug. Clearance is defined as the volume of blood completely cleared of drug per unit time, and is usually expressed as ml/min. Zero order kinetics implies that an enzyme process is saturated and therefore the metabolism of the drug will not be proportional to its concentration (as is the case in first order kinetics). This means that a small increase in dose can cause a large increase in plasma concentration for drugs such as phenytoin and ethanol.

1.   Short TG, Hood GC. Pharmacokinetics, pharmacodynamics and drug monitoring in critical illness. In: *Oh's Intensive Care Manual*, 5th Ed. Bersten AD, Soni N, Eds. Edinburgh: Butterworth Heinemann, 2003.

K96   TFFT

Fentanyl and alfentanil are both full opioid receptor agonists capable of 100% efficacy in sufficient dose. Fentanyl is more potent than alfentanil (same efficacy with a lower dose) and therefore has a dose-response curve the same shape as, but leftwards, of alfentanil. Morphine and midazolam occupy different receptors and should not be compared on the same dose-response axis. C might represent non-competitive antagonism of drug A, but flumazenil is a competitive antagonist of midazolam. The effect of flumazenil on midazolam would be better represented by line B. Line C might also represent the effect of a partial agonist compared with a full agonist (A). Buprenorphine is a partial opioid receptor agonist.

1.   Drug Action. In: *Pharmacology for Anaesthesia and Intensive Care*, 2nd Ed. Peck TE, Hill SA, Williams M, Eds. London: Greenwich Medical Media, 2003.

K97 TTFF

In a large, prospective multicentre cohort study of admissions to ICU, renal replacement therapy (RRT) was associated with a four-fold higher in-hospital mortality rate (62.8% vs. 15.6%). As well as being a marker of disease severity (i.e. associated with other factors leading to a higher risk of death), renal failure requiring RRT was shown to be an independent risk factor for death. When compared with controls matched for age and disease severity, patients requiring RRT were still far more likely to die than controls (62.8% vs. 38.5% in-hospital mortality). The leading cause of death in patients with acute renal failure is infection.

1.   Metnitz PGH, *et al.* Effect of acute renal failure requiring renal replacement therapy on outcome in critically ill patients. *Crit Care Med* 2002; 30(9): 2051-8.

K98 TTTT

Candida albicans was the most commonly isolated fungus in blood cultures in a 1-year survey of candidaemia in Scottish intensive care units (52% of cases), followed by *C. glabrata* (22.7%) [1]. In this study *C. albicans* was susceptible to a variety of antifungal agents including all those named in the question. In contrast, over 60% of isolates of *C. glabrata* were resistant to fluconazole. Treatment should be continued until 14 days after negative blood cultures have been obtained according to guidelines from the Infectious Disease Society of America [2].

1.   Odds FC, *et al.* One year prospective survey of Candida bloodstream infections in Scotland. *Journal of Medical Microbiology* 2007; 56: 1066-75.
2.   Pappas PG *et al.* Guidelines for treatment of candidiasis. *Clin Infect Dis* 2004; 38(2): 161-89.

K99 TTTT

Prone positioning of the anaesthetised patient for any length of time is associated with a variety of rare but well recognised complications. Case reports of stroke have been reported with prone positioning when the head has been rotated, presumed due to vertebral or carotid artery occlusion [1]. Weakness of hand grip, or more proximal weakness, may result from injury to the brachial plexus. This appears to be more common in patients who are positioned with one arm extended, and the risk is minimised by adducting both arms. Macroglossia and oropharyngeal swelling have been reported following operations in the prone position, probably due to increased venous pressure. This may be due in part to excessive flexion of the neck causing kinking of the internal jugular vein. Blindness is extremely rare, but may occur from retinal ischaemia secondary to raised intra-ocular pressure; this is elevated in the prone position [2] and has the effect of reducing intra-orbital perfusion pressure.

1. Lee WT, Ju CI, Kim SW. Lateral medullary syndrome caused by prone position for spine surgery. *J Korean Neurosurg Soc* 2007; 41: 118-9.
2. Ozcan MS, Praetel C, Bhatti MT, *et al*. The effect of body inclination during prone positioning on intraocular pressure in awake volunteers: a comparison of two operating tables. *Anesth Analg* 2004; 99: 1152-8.
3. Edgcombe H, Carter K, Yarrow S. Anaesthesia in the prone position. *Br J Anaesth* 2008; 100(2): 165-83.

K100 TFFF

Coma may occur as a consequence of traumatic or metabolic/hypoxic brain injury. This rarely lasts longer than a month, and may progress to any point on a spectrum between vegetative state and full recovery of higher mental function. The prognosis of persistent vegetative state (PVS) is worse for patients with a metabolic cause than those who have suffered trauma. Such patients have a <1% chance of improvement if PVS is still present at 3 months post-insult. The Glasgow Coma Scale score is of little use in the assessment of these patients who are 'awake but not aware'. Specialised scoring systems such as the Disorders of Consciousness Scale (DOCS) have been developed for this purpose. CT and MRI scans demonstrate widespread cortical and thalamic atrophy in PVS patients which progresses with time. Such imaging is of little help in prognostication, although functional MRI imaging and positron emission tomography (PET) show promise in this regard. The mortality of the PVS is estimated to be 70% at 3 years and 84% at 5 years, and may be influenced by the aggressiveness of management of complications such as pressure sores and infections.

1.   Bernat JL. Chronic disorders of consciousness. *Lancet* 2006; 367: 1181-92.